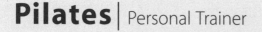

Pilates | Personal Trainer

Getting Started with **Stretching** WORKOUT

D0735257

HAGAN MEMORIAL Library
821 Walnut Street
Williamsburg, KY 40769

Pilates | Personal Trainer

Getting Started with Stretching WORKOUT

Illustrated step-by-step matwork routine

Michael King

Yolande Green

Ulysses Press

RA
781

K56
2003

Copyright © 2003 Ulysses Press. All rights reserved. No part of this publication may be reproduced, stored in a retrieval system, or transmitted in any form or by any means without the prior written permission of the publisher, nor be otherwise circulated in any form of binding or cover other than that in which it is published and without a similar condition being imposed on the subsequent purchaser.

Published in the United States by
Ulysses Press
P.O. Box 3440
Berkeley, CA 94703
www.ulyssespress.com

Published in the United Kingdom as *Pilates: The Complete Body System* (2002) and *Pure Pilates* (2000) by Mitchell Beazley, an imprint of Octopus Publishing Group Ltd

Library of Congress Card Number 2003104403
ISBN 1-56975-354-7

Printed in Canada by Transcontinental Printing

10 9 8 7 6 5 4 3 2 1

Interior Design	Kenny Grant
Cover Design	Sarah Levin
Photography	Ruth Jenkinson
Models	Beth Caterer
	Nancy Markwick
	Malcolm Muirhead
	Simon Spalding

Distributed in the United States by Publishers Group West and in Canada by Raincoast Books

Please Note
This book has been written and published strictly for informational purposes, and in no way should be used as a substitute for consultation with health care professionals. You should not consider educational material herein to be the practice of medicine or to replace consultation with a physician or other medical practitioner. The author and publisher are providing you with information in this work so that you can have the knowledge and can choose, at your own risk, to act on that knowledge. The author and publisher also urge all readers to be aware of their health status and to consult health care professionals before beginning any health program.

contents

INTRODUCTION

9   Why Pilates?

12 Holistic program

14 The workout

16 Preventing pain

VITAL ELEMENTS

20 Concentration

23 Breathing

26 Centering

31 Control

34 Posture

37 Neutral spine

40 Precision

42 Isolation

THE WORKOUT

46 Warm-up stretching

68 Strength & stretching

90 Glossary

92 Index

96 About the authors/
       Acknowledgments

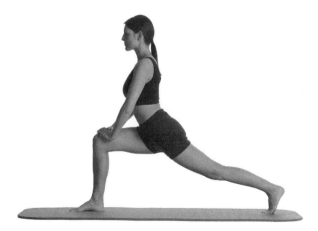

introduction

Pilates is not a fitness fad; it is a holistic concept that will not only make you feel fitter and more flexible, but will enrich your whole way of life. The series of movements will not only change how your body looks, but it will also give you a new physical poise and greater mental strength.

During my years as an exercise instructor, I have witnessed many trend shifts in the fitness industry—from high impact to low impact aerobics, from slide to step, and from spinning to core and functional training. Some of these changes have been introduced because of safety concerns over certain movements or ways of exercising. The advantage of a Pilates system, in contrast, is that the movements can be gentle on your body. The technique can also be effectively used to complement other exercise regimes.

I am one of a third generation of Pilates instructors following Joseph Pilates and writing this book is part of my effort to give others an insight into the power of the Pilates way. I would like to pass on all the information and knowledge that I have developed over my years in the fitness industry, training people in the physical skills to enrich the quality of their lives.

It is very exciting to witness the current popularity of Pilates. From the perspective of someone with a back injury who has worked with many different types of exercise, I have seen the value of the Pilates technique and the way that it changes people. You may believe that a hunched posture is part of getting older, but this is not the case. If you pay regular attention to your body and invest in it by incorporating stretching and challenging exercises into your routines, then you will benefit by feeling fitter and more attractive. You can also maintain these benefits as you grow older.

Balancing your body

Pilates is a system of exercise that, when regularly practiced, will improve your flexibility and strength. The movements will have a noticeable impact on your body in terms of general well-being, youthfulness, and flexibility, and they will also help to heal any long- or short-term injuries. Even moderate regular daily activities may result in recurring aches or physical problems. Sitting at a desk all day, for example, unbalances your body, causing the hip flexors (the front muscles of your thighs) and the upper back to form themselves into a rounded position. Pilates helps to release such tensions and ease your body back into a more natural balance. It also helps you to achieve a leaner body, feel more poised, less anxious, and stronger mentally. The moves shown here are structured with this in mind and are based on the movements that Joseph Pilates taught.

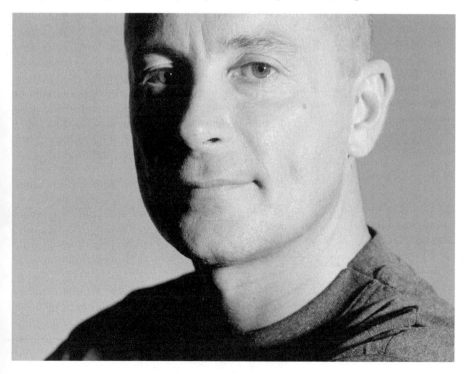

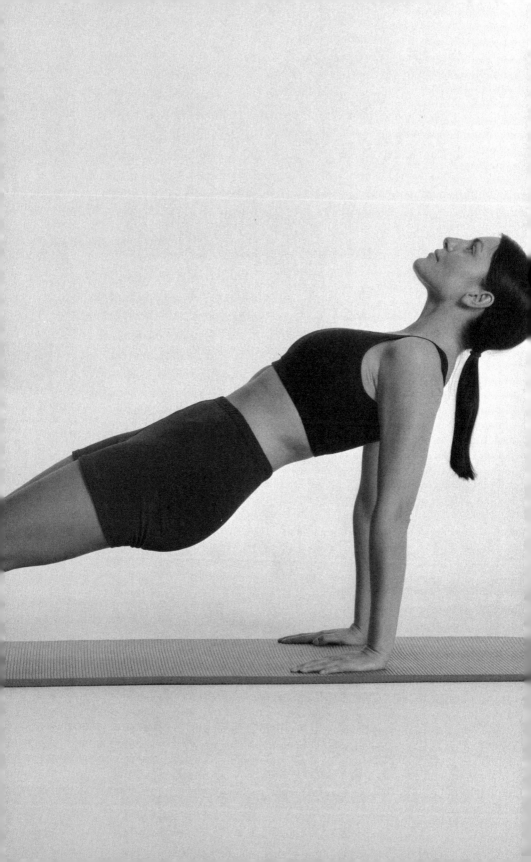

why Pilates?

The Pilates movements stretch the muscles and pull them into a longer and leaner shape, rather than forcing them to tear and rebuild into the shorter and thicker shape that conventional strength training does.

Pilates systematically exercises all the muscle groups in your body, challenging the weak areas as well as the strong. It balances the body, focuses on tight areas, and aims to increase strength and flexibility. When he conceived the original matwork exercises, Joseph Pilates was looking to stretch the body to the full to bring maximum benefit to the person exercising. Even experienced athletes may find some of his original moves difficult. This is because they use muscle control and coordination that few people are used to.

All-round benefits

The Pilates system works the body as a whole, and aims to coordinate the upper and lower muscle groups with the center of the body. This has a dramatic effect on strength, flexibility, posture, and coordination. Whether you are interested in Pilates for cosmetic, medical, or preventative reasons, the system of movements will strengthen your body and at the same time focus your mind.

Anyone can do it

You do not have to be an athlete to be involved with Pilates. And while the exercises are designed to put a minimum of strain on the body, they also aim to challenge its capabilities. This means that anyone of any age and any level of fitness can do Pilates. Whether young or old, a fitness fanatic or someone who has never exercised before, you will reap the benefits.

Basic equipment

You don't need any expensive equipment for Pilates exercises; you can follow a program at home with just a floor mat. The Pilates system is often linked to various innovative Pilates machines, equipment that can form an integral part of the exercises. However, remember that there is nothing that you can do on a machine that you can't do on the mat.

Develops concentration

Known as the intelligent way of working out, there is a focus on concentration and discipline with Pilates. Standard exercise regimes tend not to require mental discipline, but Pilates is different, healing and treating the mind and body on different levels. And because it works all the muscles in the body, simple everyday tasks such as shopping or gardening also become easier and safer.

Pilates and yoga

Pilates and Yoga have certain goals in common. Most significantly they both advocate individual progress in a non-competitive format. The exercises also share an emphasis on stretching, as well as strengthening muscles. Both Yoga and Pilates emphasize deep breathing and the use of smooth, long movements that encourage muscles to relax and lengthen. Pilates is also similar to Yoga because of the body suppleness it brings. The difference is that while some Yoga techniques involve moving from one static posture to the next without repetitions, Pilates flows through a series of movements that are more dynamic, systematic, and anatomically based.

Popular support

Although Pilates has been around since the 1920s, an understanding of this program of exercise that builds up your strength and your immune system has only become popular quite recently. Many Hollywood stars have endorsed the technique—among them Sharon Stone, Courtney Cox Arquette, Minnie Driver, Julia Roberts, and Madonna (who has even claimed that it is the only way to exercise). As a result, Pilates is no longer the domain of the rich and famous and can be practiced in most gyms and health clubs.

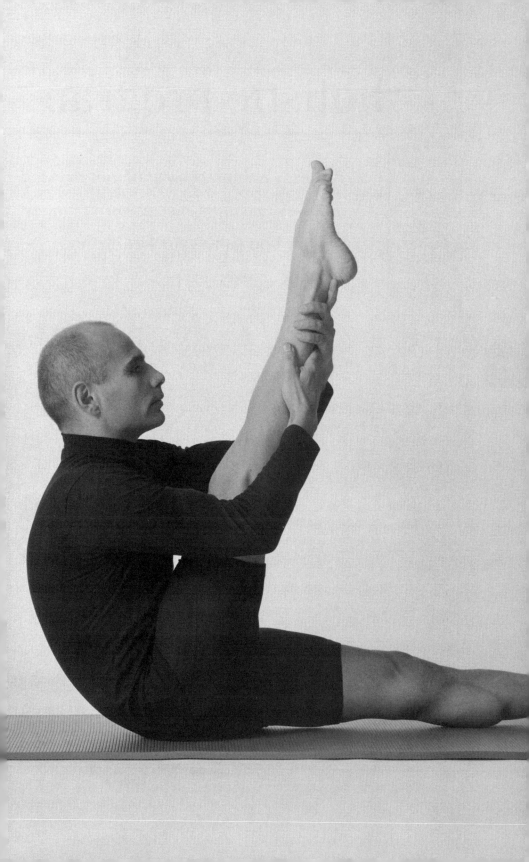

holistic program

Pilates is a thinking way of moving, and involves making a serious commitment to your body and your well-being. It is not an exercise regime to be compartmentalized in your life.

Pilates is significantly more effective when combined with enough restful sleep, a healthy diet, and a complementary fitness program. So Pilates is an invaluable, solid support system for any other regular exercise that you are involved in. It is now accepted that various fitness regimes, such as aerobics, swimming, gym work, or bodybuilding—are not inappropriate, but simply insufficient. An unbalanced exercise regime will not prepare the body for every eventuality. Even though injuries are limited in exercise classes or gyms because of thorough warming-up techniques and health-and-safety regulations, it is still common to pull muscles when lifting heavy items at home or work. What we need to adopt, and what Pilates offers, is a way of training the different parts of the body to work together, to support each other and give your body the protection that it needs.

Cross-training

Just because you have started to exercise using the Pilates method, it does not mean that you have to give up on other sports and fitness programs. On the contrary, your Pilates program is best served when it is complemented by a form of cardiovascular exercise. Complete low-stress Pilates exercises alongside aerobic ones. You will find Pilates ideal for cross-training because it will correct any postural problem associated with other forms of repetitive exercise. Pilates embraces all the areas that make up a fully integrated approach to fitness: strength, flexibility, motor skills, coordination, and relaxation.

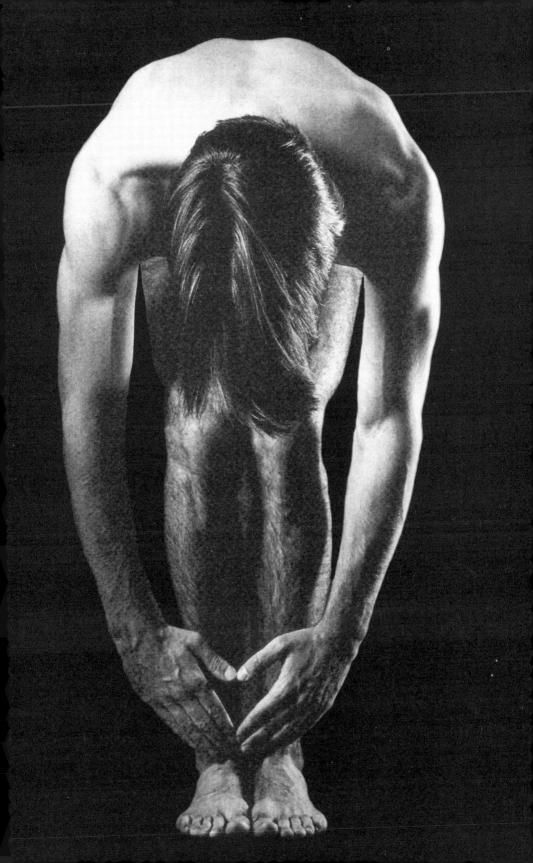

the workout

What would you like to gain from this workout? You will need to understand where your physical strengths and weaknesses lie in order to focus on exercises that will benefit you most.

Weaknesses do not only signify a lack of muscular strength, but also relate to tight areas of your body that hold you back from fully performing a task. Remember, an inflexible body will result in the same problems as one with no muscular strength.

You will find that the exercises you least enjoy are generally those your body needs to spend more time on. In the same way, those that are easier will need to be practiced less.

The workout in this book is in no way meant to replace your holistic fitness program, nor substitute for a general Pilates regimen. I have designed this back strengthening workout as a supplemental workout to address your weakness

in this one area. When added to your regular workout program, it can help bring your body into better balance.

Pure Pilates

Joseph Pilates' original book featured a series of 34 movements. I present many of these pure Pilates exercises, along with beginner variations of the moves, in my book *Pilates Workbook*. Although I would like all my students to be able to undertake the full range of these movements, as a responsible fitness leader I need to work around their capabilities.

Joseph Pilates developed his technique from instinct, and although the basic principles always remained the same, when he worked with particular students he adapted the moves according to their requirements.

So, an essential part of Pilates is knowing what you *cannot* do.

Always listen to your body, both when exercising and once you have finished, and be sensitive to any vulnerable areas.

Pacing yourself

Undertaking advanced moves at the beginning of a Pilates program is unwise. The original Pilates moves are advanced and inappropriate for those unfamiliar with the correct techniques. If you challenge yourself with Pilates exercises that are beyond your level or are uncomfortable, you then risk possible injury. If you stay sensitively attuned to your body and gradually challenge yourself, you can then move toward your ultimate goals at an effective pace.

Note: The moves in this book are at a beginner level, with intermediate variations for you to do as you get stronger.

Challenge yourself

Remember that over the long run you should equally balance both strength and mobility while working across the full range of body movements. However, starting with flexibility and light strength exercises is a good way to begin challenging yourself. This is important in order to prepare your body and enable it to perform the more demanding Pilates movements.

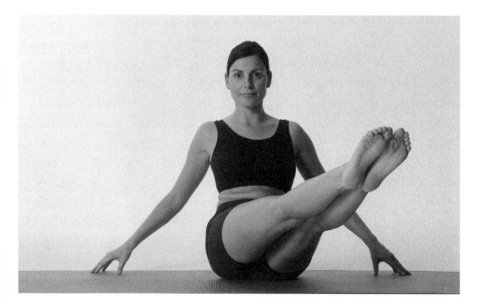

preventing pain

Even the most healthy person may have minor pains that indicate stresses and strains on the body. Never ignore these symptoms, but use them to identify which areas need more strengthening or more stretching and mobility.

Pilates trains the body to prevent injury and to maintain good posture and movement. In order to have good posture, you need to develop good muscle balance. Indeed, injuries are often related in some way to bad posture or muscular imbalances. These types of problems can occur for many reasons. Repetitive movements can be one cause, such as when a golfer continuously practices his swing on one side of the body or when someone spends long periods of time working at a desk. In fact, any pattern that destabilizes your body's natural balance and makes it tense, can lead to weakness, tightness, and a resulting danger of injury.

Pain and Gain

There is always a certain amount of discomfort that arises during training, especially when it comes to stretching muscles that you may not have used in some time. A strong stretch may elicit some pain, but be careful not to push yourself too far. If any pain is sudden or sharp you must stop immediately. This extreme should never be experienced. I emphasize again that Pilates should be performed gradually. It is always better to build up slowly. Only in this way can you strike a balance between achievement and challenge. Never exercise when you are in chronic pain or when any of your muscles are inflamed.

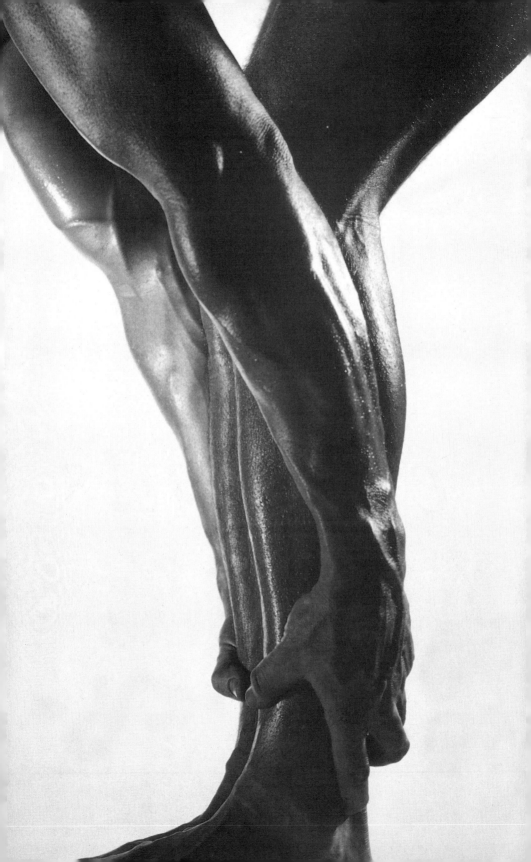

vital elements

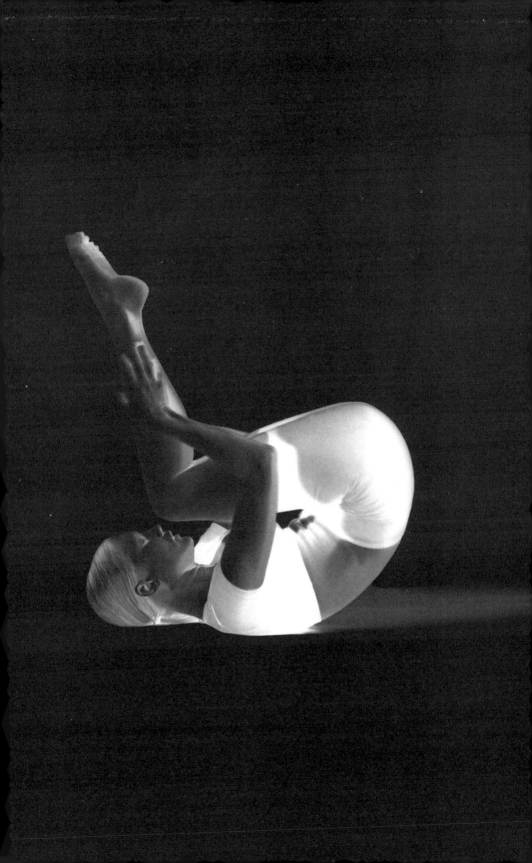

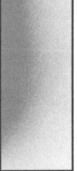

concentration

With many exercise classes and techniques you don't have to think about what you're doing, you just do it to get through it. But with Pilates, every movement is a conscious act controlled by the power of your mind.

"Always keep your mind wholly concentrated on the purpose of the exercises as you perform them." Joseph Pilates

Pilates is "the thinking way of moving" and requires a different kind of concentration than that typically used for other exercise forms. It may not be all that important to concentrate during an aerobics class or when walking on a treadmill, but it is absolutely essential for Pilates.

Setting the mood

There are simple things you can do to improve concentration. Check that the space you plan to use for Pilates is free of distractions and that it is warm and comfortable. Make sure you will not be disturbed.

Though Pilates is not a spiritual workout, you will find it very relaxing because concentrating on a single movement causes everything else that is going on in your life to fade away.

If you want to use music in the background, make sure it isn't punctuated by a heavy beat. Don't make the mistake I once made

Our inner voice

Controlling our thoughts, much like controlling our actions, is not as easy as it might first appear to be. When you are under pressure, your thoughts can become very erratic and spin off in random directions. If you are stressed, going to sleep can be especially difficult because you are unable to "switch off." Unwelcome thoughts pop into your head despite your best efforts.

Effective concentration is a skill we acquire as children. By the time we are adults, we all have a little "inner voice" that controls our actions.

First attempts at unfamiliar movements may feel strange and awkward. It is very easy to fall into the trap of performing only the moves you enjoy, when what you need most is to do the ones you do not like. Normally people speed up the difficult part of the movement to get it over with as soon as they can. Instead, you need to slow down. Only by concentrating on what you are doing can you properly control your actions.

when I used a tape of nature sounds that featured screeching parrots and mating whales!

A clear mind

You'll soon find that the benefits of practicing concentration—easier mental focus, clarity of thought, and, most importantly, reduction of stress—are well worth the effort.

All too often in our whirlwind modern lives visual clutter and noisy distractions make it difficult to focus on the task at hand. Stress itself makes concentration more difficult but persevere; mental focus is an art that improves with practice. Marshalling your powers of concentration helps you feel calmer and in control.

Making time for Pilates

Because concentration is linked to focusing on priorities, it is also needed when you are planning your exercises. Start with small sessions of 20–30 minutes, and aim to work up to an hour. It is better to have 20 minutes of a rewarding workout than an hour simply going through the motions of a routine.

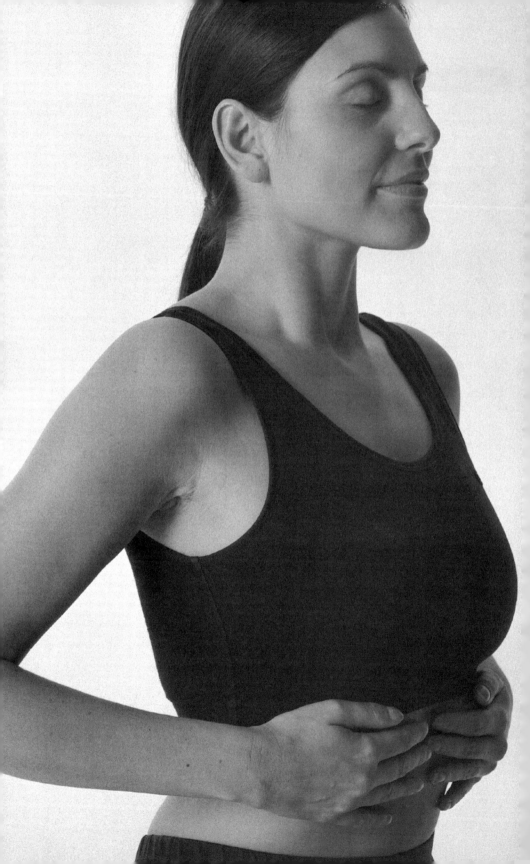

breathing

Pilates uses a controlled and continuous way of breathing that takes time to perfect, but results in a stronger and more energy-efficient body.

"Breathing is the first act of life. Our very life depends on it. Millions have never learned to master the art of correct breathing."

Joseph Pilates

As babies and young children, we breathe correctly, but as adults we tend to develop poor breathing patterns. Correct breathing ensures a good flow of oxygen to the working muscles, which then cleanses the bloodstream and energizes the whole body. Breathing also improves concentration and aids smooth and fluid movement.

There are many types of breathing techniques, and different types can make movements easier, harder, or more controlled. A correct breathing technique can be mastered, but it takes time and patience.

So how should we breathe?

In Pilates, we follow a breath called thoracic or lateral breathing. This means breathing wide and full into your back and sides, opening the ribcage as you breathe. Think of your lungs as bellows, expanding and widening as you breathe in and closing down as you breathe out. This way of breathing works the intercostal muscles, the muscles between the ribs. When these muscles are working, the upper body is more mobile and fluid in its movements.

Pilates exercises are designed in combination with breathing techniques to work the correct muscles to create the required movement. The core muscles always support this process.

Normal breathing

When you inhale normally, the lungs expand, the diaphragm drops and the stomach moves out. As you exhale, your diaphragm lifts and the stomach moves in. This is called "abdominal" breathing and is quite natural.

The wrong way

Whatever you do, don't hold your breath. Most people hold their breath if they pick up something heavy, much as weightlifters would when picking up a barbell. This type of breathing is called the Valsalvic method and results in a stressful increase in blood pressure. It wastes energy in parts of the body where it isn't required. In Pilates you want to keep your breathing continuous.

Muscles that make up the core

The following groups of muscles make up your core or center.

- *TA (transverse abdominal) muscles* are the corset-like muscles that wrap around the center of your body.
- *Multifidus muscles* run down the length of the spine. They link two or three vertebrae and can create or block movement.
- *The pelvic floor* is the sling muscle that runs from the front of the pelvis to the lower part of the spine.
- *The diaphragm* is the muscle that lies under the ribcage and helps you to inhale and exhale.

Thoracic breathing exercise

Sit comfortably or stand tall. Place your hands on the front of your ribcage with your fingertips just touching. As you breathe in, fill the lungs, open the ribcage, and let the fingers slide apart. As you breathe out, let them slide back to touch again. This can take considerable practice. To advance the exercise, move your hands farther around so that your hands are touching your armpits, and breathe to push your ribcage into your hands. If you can reach, extend your palms around to your back.

Another option is to place both hands on the front of the ribcage and breathe first into the right hand, then into the left hand, then into both hands equally. This will increase your body awareness and your breathing control.

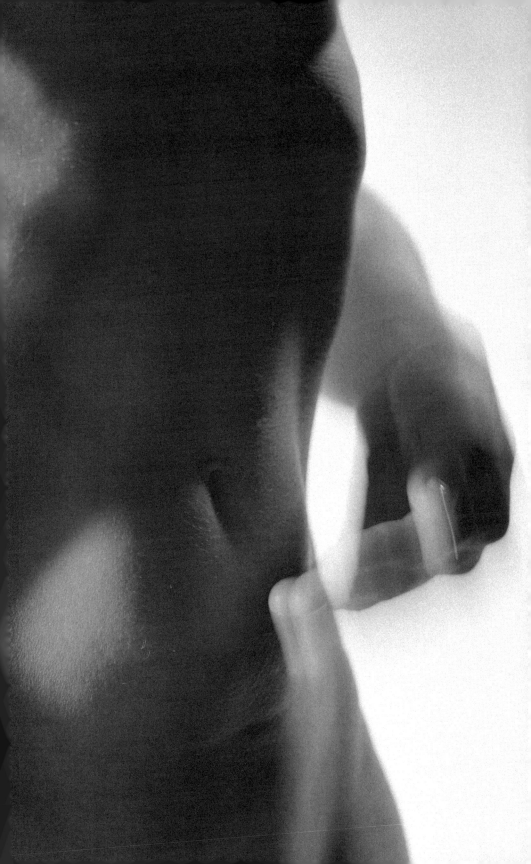

centering

The body is designed to work as a complete unit. If you train to do this, you will have a solid center to create the physical power for each movement. In order to visualize the body as an integrated unit, think of a conductor bringing together all the sections of an orchestra to perform a concerto.

Joseph Pilates believed that our abdominal muscles, now known as abs, function as the "powerhouse" for the whole of the body. Your abs are your center and they initiate every movement. To maintain a strong center you need an equal balance of strength between the abs and the back.

The core

We have already referred to the core (see breathing on page 23) as consisting of four muscle groups: the TA muscles, the multifidus muscles (back muscles), the pelvic floor muscles, and the diaphragm.

Imagine your core as a tree trunk, the core being the solid supporting center of your arms, legs, and head. If you imagine cutting through the tree trunk, the muscles of your body represent the rings of age in the tree: The global muscles (the rectus abdominus muscle) are on the outside of the trunk. As you move toward the center you'll find the external oblique muscles, the internal oblique muscles, and finally the TA muscles.

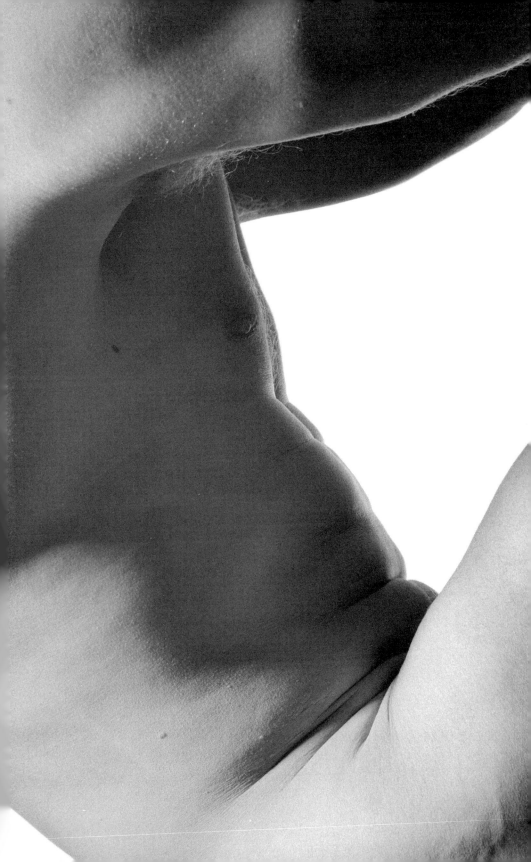

30 percent contraction

Every exercise is controlled or initiated from the contraction of two of the core muscles, the TA muscles or the pelvic floor. This is because these muscles help to stabilize the body as you move.

For many years, Pilates practitioners would pull in the lower abdominal muscles tighter as the movement became more challenging. Now, however, research has established that this is not the most effective way to work these muscles. Drawing in the abdominal muscles as hard as you can activates the core muscles with what I call 100 percent effort. This tires the muscles quickly, and it does not train them to operate effectively in everyday activities. Research has shown that the most effective way to train them is at 30 percent of their maximum strength. This allows them to be used throughout an hour's session without causing fatigue. They will also become naturally stronger and support you as you perform your daily activities. Work through the following exercises to help you to find your center.

Pelvic floor and TA muscles

Activate your center either through the TA muscles (shown opposite) or by using the pelvic floor muscles. Research has shown that it is not productive to use both muscles together, so when following your routine, try to activate your center by using only one group of muscles.

Activating the TA muscles

Imagine that you have a belt around your waist and that the abdominal muscles draw in when you tighten it. Use the images on page 29 (stages 1–3) to establish the most efficient level at which to perform the exercises.

Activating the pelvic floor

The pelvic floor runs from the front of the pelvis to the lower spine and supports you like a sling. This is one of the hardest muscles to activate, but when mastered it will be easy to practice wherever you are without anyone knowing. You can activate the pelvic floor muscle by imagining that you are trying to stop your urine in mid-flow.

Imagine that your pelvic floor is the floor of an elevator. As you breathe out, draw up the elevator as far as you can to the tenth floor. Then release this halfway to the fifth floor and then a little farther to the third floor. This is the level of exertion that you want to follow in the program. Continue the exercise with the following pattern: move the elevator to the tenth floor, return to the ground floor, up again to the fifth floor, and back to the ground floor. Finally go up to the third floor and back down. When you do this exercise, you can be sitting or standing—the key is to be comfortable.

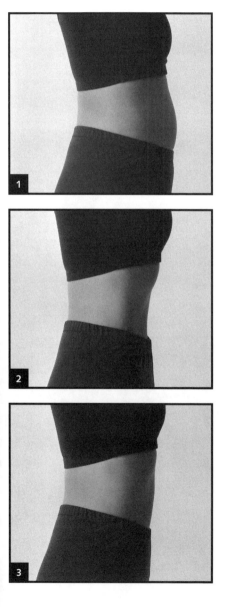

1 In a standing position, allow your abdominal muscles to relax and form a dome. Don't push them out. Instead, become aware of how the rest of your body feels as you release these muscles.

2 As you breathe out, draw in the abdominal muscles as far as you can. Imagine that a belt is being tightened around you, that it will be tightened right up to the last notch. This is what I call 100 percent effort.

3 Relax the muscles halfway to reach the "fifth notch" on the belt. Think of this as 50 percent effort. Then release them a little more to the "third notch," or 30 percent effort. This is the level at which to work efficiently throughout your program.

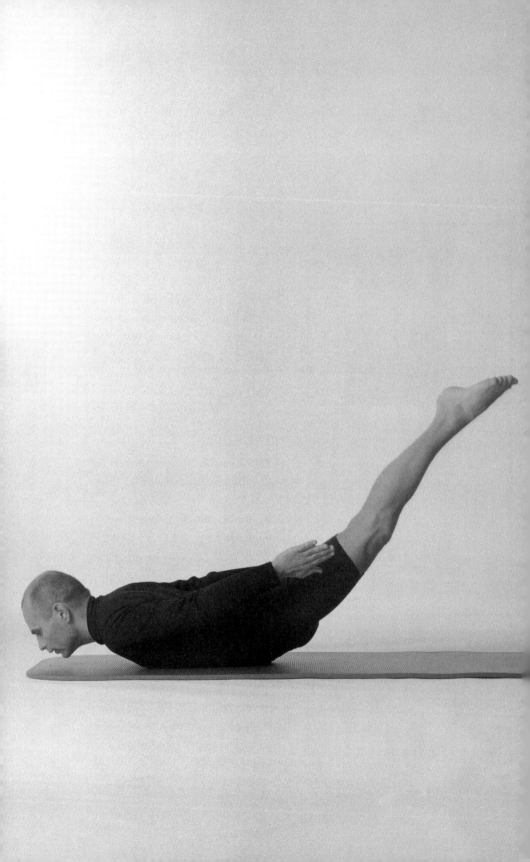

control

Good posture can be achieved only when the body is under perfect control. When doing the exercises, aim for slow, studied movements, and allow them to flow from start to finish to form a continuous sequence. Continue in this way until you have completed the total number of repetitions.

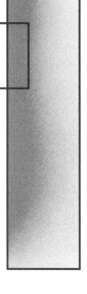

Working with the weight of your body against the natural pull of gravity requires considerable control. In fact, we are all accustomed to controlling our bodies: the process of walking is not a haphazard series of movements, but rather a controlled sequence that we have learned from childhood. However, many of us, quite unconsciously, developed bad habits in the way that we move that may later affect our physical health.

Maintaining control means ensuring that the body moves with purpose and direction at all times. A controlled movement involves making the relevant muscles and joints work to their full capacity while at the same time not wasting any energy. This concept is integral to the philosophy of Pilates.

Pilates exercises strengthen the body, and the slower and more controlled the movements, the greater the strength you gain from them.

Visualization

The use of visual associations can be effective when working with

Pilates. Visualization can help you understand how to control your movements and also how to gain the most from your workouts.

For example, I have already noted that Pilates exercises need to be continuous, to flow from one stage to another freely, without interruption. So, if you are trying a new movement, it might be helpful to think, as you begin, of a Ferris wheel at a fairground—the wheel turning slowly and deliberately. Or,

think of a tightrope walker at the circus. In order to stay on the rope she has to maintain perfect control of her body, to move slowly and deliberately from one end of the rope to the other. Such visualizations are used throughout this book to give you deeper insight into how each exercise should feel.

The powerhouse

In disciplines such as tai chi, it is believed that the powerhouse is the store of the *chi*, or life energy. With physical movements, the energy is generated from the powerhouse, then carried to the relevant part of the body to give it power. This is equivalent to the core or center in Pilates.

Graceful control

When practicing Pilates, make every movement as smooth and graceful as you can. To use a visualization, imagine that you are a dancer performing a movement on a stage in front of an audience you want to impress with your grace and poise.

Think, too, about every part of your body as you move. Does each part have an important role in the execution of the movement, and are both sides of your body

Resist me

Find a partner. Stand up, holding a towel in your right hand. Have your partner sit down at your feet and hold the other end of the towel with both hands. Pull your fist, with the towel, toward your shoulder in a bicep curl. Let your partner create resistance so that there is equal tension as you move your arm up and down.

Think about a resistance scale from one to ten. One is when your partner exerts no resistance with the towel. Ten is when your partner pulls so hard that you can't move at all. Aim for a resistance level of five in both directions. Breathe out as you curl the arm up and breathe in as you uncurl the muscle. Repeat 10 times and change arms.

Next, drop the towel but imagine you are still holding it and repeat the bicep curl. Do you feel the resistance that you had when you were holding the towel? This technique will aid controlled action.

Slower is harder

Begin by doing five regular push-ups, either with your legs fully extended in the full push-up position, or with your knees on the floor (the three-quarter position). Do these first five at your normal pace.

Now do another five, but count two slow counts down and two slow counts up. Breathe in as you go down and out as you come up. Rest. Now repeat, but to a count of four in each direction. Rest. Finally, try a last five push-ups, to a count of six on the way down and another six on the way up, without pausing at the top or at the bottom, making all five push-ups one long, continuous, and steady movement. It was harder than you thought, wasn't it?

At this latter point you are working at the same intensity that you should be working at while doing the Pilates exercises. Pilates is all about quality and range of movement, with the contraction of the muscles (the downward movement in this case) and the flexion (the pushing up movement) requiring equal effort.

working at the same level? If not, rebalance yourself so that each part has an equal role.

Full range

This type of movement can be applied to other forms of exercise with much success: try using resistance machines or free weights in the gym with slow, steady, and even movements. You will be able to feel the difference and the exercises will prove more effective (you may have to use a lighter weight).

It is also vitally important to ensure that you are using your full range of movement. Check that you are working equally hard, with the same intensity and resistance throughout. As much effort should be used to extend a muscle (eccentric movement) as to contract it (concentric movement). By working in this way, you will begin to develop strength and flexibility in equal measure, giving your muscles (and your body) a long, lean look.

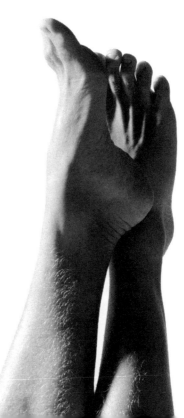

posture

Good posture is vital. Having bad posture will prevent your body from functioning efficiently, and it will also undermine your balance and coordination. The danger is that if you develop a habit of having bad posture, your body will accept it as normal and will learn to suffer any associated aches and pains.

An ideal posture will have all the joints in a neutral position so that they are without stress. The joint will follow the natural alignment of the bones. A neutral position will reduce wear on the joints, promote balance, and keep the muscles around the joints in correct alignment. This in turn allows the internal organs to feel comfortable and function efficiently. It is important that you establish a neutral position before you start each exercise.

Poor posture

Poor posture can lead to many adverse symptoms, which include:

- *Fatigue*
- *Neck and shoulder tension*
- *Headaches*
- *Impaired balance and coordination*
- *Muscular weakness*
- *Poor circulation*
- *Tension and stress*
- *Digestive problems*
- *Aching and painful joints*

Correcting poor posture

There are the three main types of problematic posture: sway-back (see stage 1), lordorsis (see stage 2), and kyphosis (rounding of the shoulders or hunching). It is also possible to have a combination of these postures.

Poor posture can be corrected, but it will take time and patience. As well as realignment exercises, you will need to give your body time to adjust to a different position. Some bad postures can be corrected surprisingly quickly while others need more time to fix.

The plumbline test

Assess your posture in front of a full-length mirror, wearing just your underwear. Stand in profile, and turn your head to the mirror.

Imagine a plumbline hanging from your ear and look at the joints that the line runs through. With a healthy posture, the line should run through the ear lobe, the center of the neck, the tip of the shoulder, the center of the ribcage, slightly behind the hip joint, the center of the knee joint, and just in front of the anklebone.

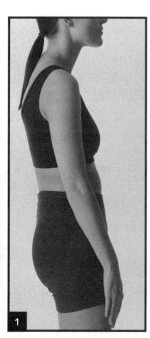

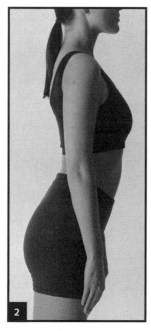

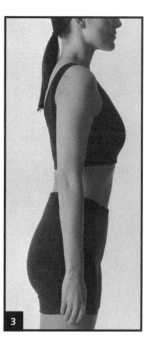

1 Sway-back posture, often called the slouch position, is common among teenagers.

2 The lordotic posture is characterized by an increased curve in the lower part of the spine.

3 With an ideal posture, gravity is evenly distributed and all joints are in their neutral position.

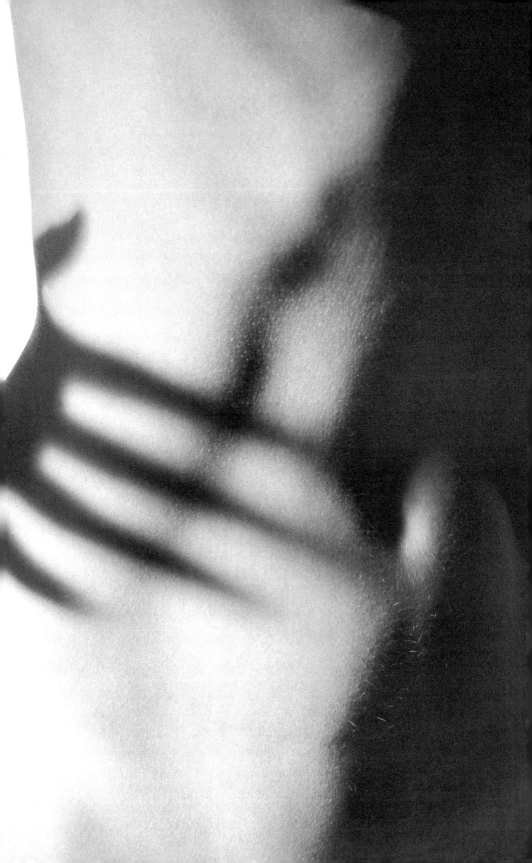

neutral spine

A neutral spine is used to describe when your spine is in its most natural position. This will not necessarily be the position that feels most comfortable. It is quite likely that your "normal" posture has been created by poor habits and you have become accustomed to the way it feels.

Finding a position with a neutral spine can be a real challenge. It is essential, however, that you find your neutral position and sustain it before undertaking any Pilates moves. Once you have started the exercises that follow, you will need to learn to hold the neutral position as your body is moving.

Training out of neutral

If your body loses the correct neutral position as you exercise the benefit to you is lost. In this scenario, you are simply making your body stronger in your preferred, non-neutral position, one that has been created by bad habits. Training in a non-neutral position also increases your chances of acquiring muscular imbalances, injuries, and increasing tension because your body is not adequately supported.

Pelvis and spine

While it is important that *all* your joints are in neutral during the moves, this section focuses on the pelvis and spine. The position of the pelvis and the position of the lower spine always affect each other. If your pelvis is rolled forward, for example, the curve in your lower spine will be exaggerated, and will not form a neutral position.

Finding neutral

You should always practice finding neutral either by lying down or by standing—the principle is the same—before starting any exercises. Most people find that lying down is the easier way to start because the floor provides some support. Follow the stages described below to find neutral.

Stage one

This stage shows the spine out of neutral with an increased lower spine curve. Start by lying on the floor in a relaxed position with your knees bent and your feet flat on the floor. Softly tilt the pelvis forward so that the space under your lower back increases. Be careful not to push this position too far because it may cause discomfort in your lower spine. See how each part of your body—particularly your legs, chest, and arms—feels in this position. Then relax back out of the position.

Stage two

The second picture shows the spine out of neutral with no lower spine curve. In the same lying position, softly tilt your pelvis back

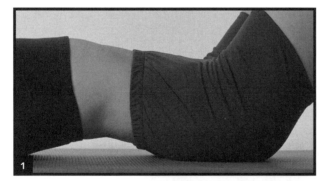

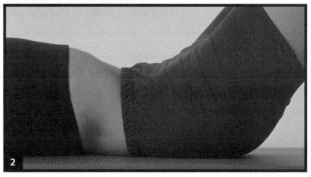

and visualize imprinting your lower spine into the mat. Don't push this position too far, and stop if it feels uncomfortable. Notice how each part of your body—particularly your legs, abdominal muscles, back, and waist—feels in this position. Then relax back out of the position.

Stage three

The third picture shows the spine in neutral. To find this position, shift your body between stages one and two, and find a position halfway between the two points. This should leave a small space under your lower back. Notice how each part of your body feels in this position—there should be no tension in the legs, chest, or back.

Stage four

The fourth stage shows the clock technique, another way to help find neutral.

Place your hands on your lower abdominal muscles with your little fingers pointing down toward your pubic bone. Imagine that your hands are a clockface (with the fingers pointing to 12 o'clock and your thumbs pointing to 6 o'clock). Tilt the pelvis forward and backward, so that 12 o'clock is higher, then 6 o'clock is higher. Neutral is the position where 12 o'clock and 6 o'clock are level.

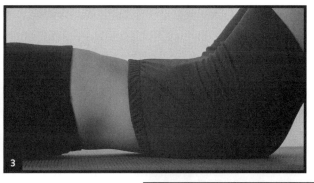

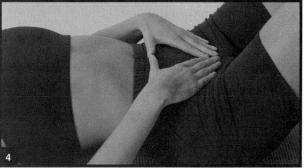

precision

You have your own natural geometry. Pilates can help you move with more precision and discover for yourself the dimensions of natural grace.

All Pilates movements are exact, and involve precise actions and precise breathing. When you think of precision and movement, you might think of synchronized swimmers or the exacting choreography that dancers can achieve. Joseph Pilates trained as both a boxer and an acrobatic circus performer, which gave him an appreciation of precision skills as well as an acute awareness of space and time.

Perfect reach

Bring to mind the image of the spread-eagled figure drawn by Leonardo da Vinci. The artist drew a circle around the figure as he stretched out to his fullest extent. These lines of geometry are a useful visualization of the space around us. Or, imagine the arm of a ballet dancer arching like the tip of a compass; we are all capable of making similar pin points in space.

You are usually unaware of the space you occupy and how your movements take place within it. Because Pilates demands that you move and breathe correctly, you will become more aware, through concentration and the use of precision, of how your personal space is created. It is through precision that you can attain graceful movement.

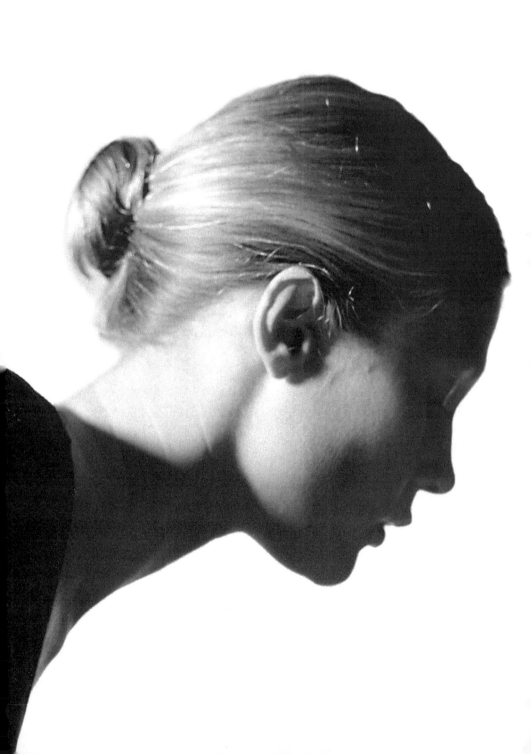

isolation

The Pilates technique is an excellent way of educating yourself and understanding, through movement, how your body works, in part and as a whole. Harmony comes from the integration of isolated parts.

"Each muscle may cooperatively and loyally aid in the uniform development of all our muscles." Joseph Pilates

For many years exercise teachers have talked about isolating different muscles. Yet it is only theoretically possible to see them in isolation; in practice, your muscles work together in groups. Often, in regular exercise classes focus has been on "spot reducing" certain areas to achieve a desired look. But in doing this you develop one muscle at the expense of another. Consequently, the whole balance of the body is thrown out of kilter. This "lopsided" approach is altogether at odds with the logic of the Pilates method.

Muscle balance

So, when we talk about isolation in Pilates we are simply making sure that you identify all your muscles for yourself, especially the weaker ones. Pilates exercises ensure you develop the neglected areas of the body that work alongside opposing, stronger muscles. For example, if you are a golfer, you know that when you play, you only

Touch and visualize

Sit down on a chair with a dumbbell, bag of sugar, or bottle of water to use as a weight. Sitting upright, hold the weight above your head in the right hand, with your right arm stretched straight toward the ceiling. Bring the left hand up to touch the back of your upper right arm with the tips of your fingers, keeping your right elbow close to your head. Lower the weight slightly behind your head and lift it back again to the ceiling. With the fingers of your left hand feel the tricep muscle at the back of the arm contracting and extending. Repeat 10–20 times. Now shift the weight to the other hand and repeat.

Finally, repeat the movement without the weight and without touching the triceps. From what you have just experienced, try and visualize the muscle working.

stronger you will remain proportionally imbalanced.

Try the "Touch and visualize" exercise (see box) to better understand how your muscles work. Learn to identify the location of, say, your tricep without actually having to touch it. Visualization techniques help you connect mentally with the muscle. Over time you will be able to feel and identify various muscles working in combination as you perform the movements.

swing in one direction. Over a period of time your body then becomes over-trained in this direction. Although not all of us play golf, we all harbor muscle imbalances to some degree. It is not uncommon to discover these over- or under-trained areas through Pilates.

Weak links

Try to be aware of any imbalance in muscle strength or flexibility as you perform the movements. Your goal here is to work toward strengthening the weaker of the two sets of muscles so that balance is regained. Otherwise, as you get

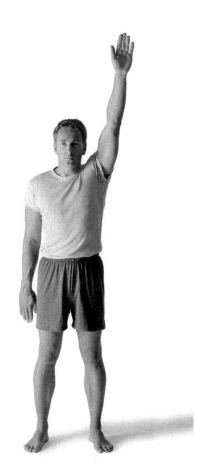

workout

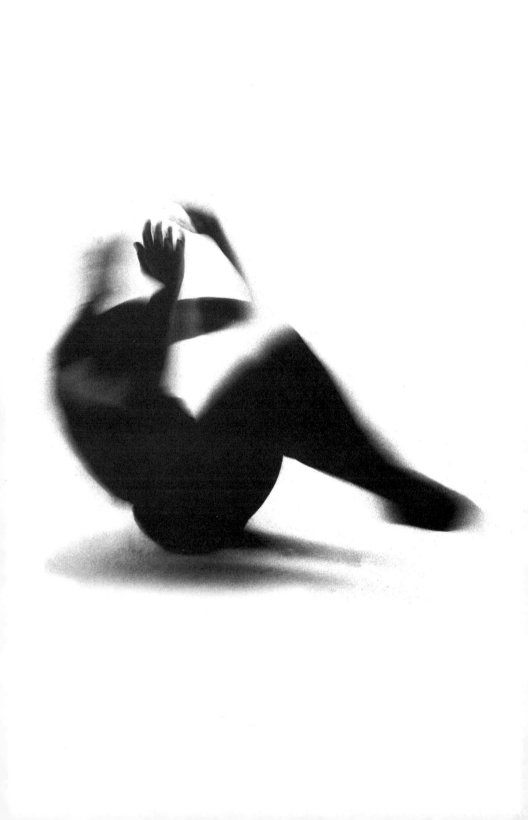

warm-up stretching

The warm-up stretches are designed to mobilize, lengthen, and stretch the muscles in preparation for more demanding movements. Use them to familiarize yourself with how your body feels as it moves and to focus on your breathing and posture before moving on to the main exercises.

wall stretch

█ CAUTION

Don't lock your elbows, and make sure that the surface you are leaning against is strong.

reps	5 breaths each side
visual cue	hand glued to wall
emphasis	top of chest

1 Stand with your left side to the wall. Place your left hand on the wall, then take a small step forward with both feet. Maintain a neutral spine, but with your feet close together. As you breathe out, lean slightly forward. Hold the stretch for one breath, then release the stretch. Repeat 5 times.

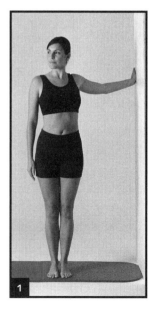

standing chest stretch

This exercise is aimed at stretching the major muscles of the chest called the pectorals. Stand tall in a neutral position and think about lengthening up and through the chest and the ribcage.

reps	5–10 breaths
visual cue	on parade
emphasis	stretch

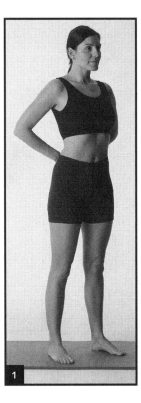

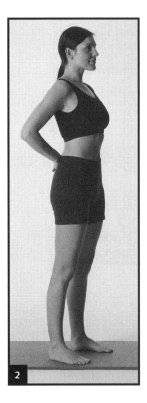

1 Stand tall in a neutral position with your feet hip-width apart. Place your palms on your lower back with your hands comfortably close to each other. Concentrate on maintaining a neutral position and not forcing the lower back out of neutral.

2 As you breathe out, try to draw the elbows closer together. As you do this, open the chest, stand tall, and keep your eyes looking forward and slightly lifted as if looking over the horizon.

round back (the cat)

WORKOUT

This movement will release your back.

! CAUTION

Begin with small movements and gradually allow them to build in size. Do not force the movement and always keep your abs tucked in.

reps	10 times
visual cue	cat stretch
emphasis	mobility

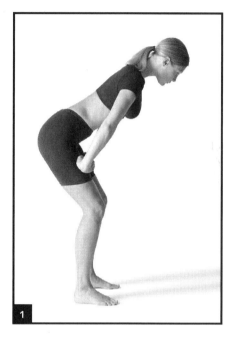

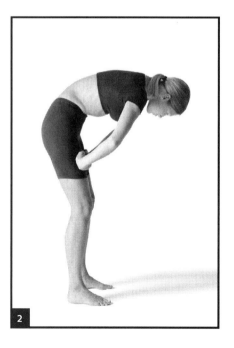

1 Put your hands on your thighs and lengthen your spine by stretching your head and neck diagonally upward. Your tail bone should curl away from you. Pull in your abs and let your shoulder blades slide down your back.

2 Breathe out and gently round your back. Imagine a string attached to your waistband, pulling you up and backward. Repeat the warm-up without stopping; keep working in a single continuous movement. Breathe in as you return to the starting position and be sure to avoid hollowing your back in the opposite direction.

swinging

This movement will warm up your spine and back muscles. Be gentle with yourself and do not force the body. Move slowly and with control, as if you were moving through water.

reps	20 times
visual cue	low bow
emphasis	mobility

1 With your feet apart and knees relaxed, stretch your arms straight up to the ceiling. Pull in your abs.

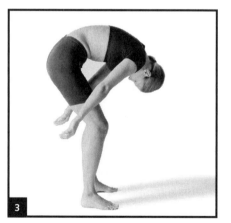

2 Breathe out and let your arms fall forward past your head. As they swing, allow your knees to bend and your back to curve. Relax your head and shoulders and pay attention to your spine as it gently relaxes, curling over. Keep your abs tight and the movement gentle.

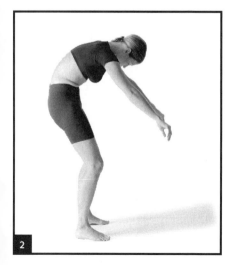

3 After reaching the curled position, breathe in and roll slowly back up to the standing position. Each time you repeat the movement, try to stretch a little farther toward the ceiling. Imagine a string is attached to the top of your head, pulling your entire body upward.

standing spine twist

Concentrate on lengthening and maintaining the third notch on the belt (see page 29). As you rotate, focus on keeping your hips facing forward with both feet planted on the ground, rather than allowing the hips to rotate with you.

reps	5–10 times each side
visual cue	corkscrew
emphasis	spine mobility

1 Standing tall in the neutral position, place the hands together in a praying gesture. Softly draw the shoulder blades back and then down into a soft "V." The thumbs should be placed on the sternum. Keep the thumbs there throughout the exercise so that the movement involves more than the arms. Take a breath in to prepare yourself.

2 As you breathe out, slowly rotate to the right, keeping the thumbs on the sternum and the nose in line with the thumbs. Focus on moving from the area between the shoulder blades. The whole center column should rotate as a single unit; don't let the head or arms rotate on their own. As you breathe in, rotate back to the center. On the next outbreath, rotate to the left, then back to the center as you breathe in. When rotating, allow your breathing rate to control the speed of the movement. Try to lengthen your spine a little farther each time you rotate back to the center.

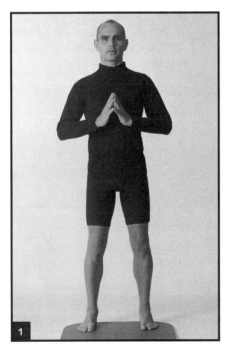

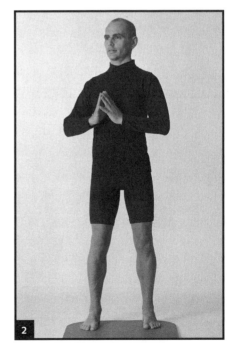

spine swing

Try not to overrotate the movement from the hips; instead, maintain the length in your lower spine. Keep the shoulders drawn down into the soft "V" and the belt muscle on the third notch (see page 29).

reps	5–10 times each side
visual cue	trailing hands
emphasis	spine mobility

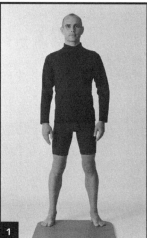

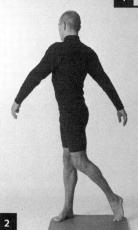

1 Stand tall with the spine in the neutral position and the feet slightly farther apart than the hips. Breathe in to prepare yourself.

2 As you breathe out, slowly rotate to the right, allowing the left heel to lift slightly. Keep the arms relaxed beside you and your knees soft and relaxed. Allow your head to turn to look over your shoulder.

3 Breathe in and rotate to the other side, keeping the movement continuously flowing with no breaks in the middle. The arms are relaxed and the heels lift naturally as you rotate.

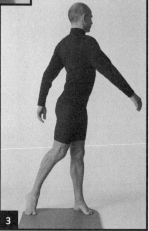

balance 1

As you breathe out, slowly lift the leg. If you would like to challenge yourself, keep the leg lifted for 2–5 breaths before lowering it.

reps	5 times each side
visual cue	tightrope
emphasis	balance

1 Stand tall in the neutral position and keep your eyes focused on a point in front of you as if you are looking toward the horizon. Keep your hips as still as possible and lengthen out your right toe in front of you, keeping the toe in contact with the floor. The hips should be still, shoulder blades drawn down into a soft "V," and the arms relaxed beside you. The belt muscle should be on the third notch (see page 29).

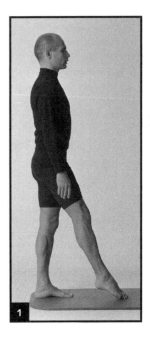

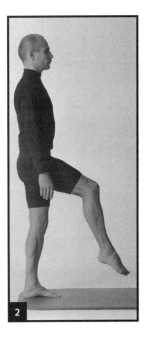

2 As you breathe out, slowly lift the right foot off the floor with the knee bent and the foot relaxed. Concentrate on keeping the left knee slightly bent, the hips still, and the weight even in the left foot. Imagine three points on the sole of your left foot: one under the big toe, one under the little toe, and one under the heel. Aim to keep an even pressure across all three points.

balance 2

Keep the weight evenly distributed across the left foot in the same way as the previous balance exercise. Be sure that the supporting knee remains soft.

reps	5 times each side
visual cue	tightrope
emphasis	balance

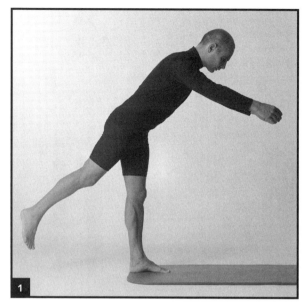

1

1 Starting from the neutral position, breathe out and lengthen the right leg and right arm. Don't lift the leg too high and lean slightly forward to allow the spine to remain lengthened and neutral. Keep the eyes looking down so that the neck stays in a neutral position.

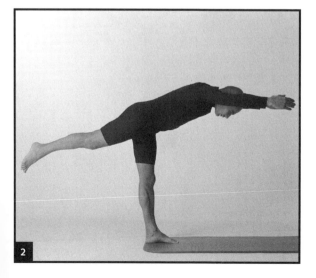

2

2 Keep lengthening through the movement until you reach a position where you feel you can maintain the balance and a neutral spine. Think about lengthening along the whole of the spine, from the head to the tailbone. As you breathe in, with control, reverse the movement to finish in a tall, standing position.

chest stretch

This movement warms up the chest muscles. Do not reach the same point each time but try and spread your arms farther. Visualize that you are creating space in the joints.

reps	10 times
visual cue	"V" shape
emphasis	mobility

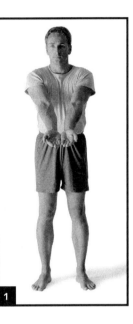

1 Stand tall with your feet apart, knees soft, and your arms stretched out with palms up in front of you. Breathe in.

2 Breathe out and stretch your arms up and to the sides. Keep your spine long by pulling that invisible string attached to the top of your head toward the ceiling. As you open your arms check that you are contracting your abs. Do not let your back arch. Keep the movement slow and the speed constant, returning to the start position.

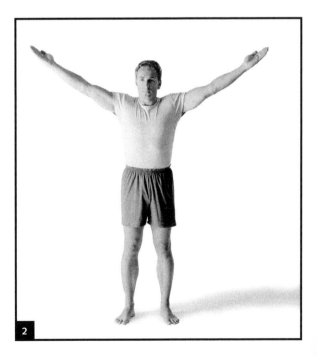

one-arm circles

This movement opens up the shoulder joints.

█ CAUTION

Do not lock your elbows and always work within your limits. If you find that you are able to make bigger circles on one side than the other, work on the weaker side in order to achieve balance in the body.

reps	10 times each side
visual cue	drawing circles
emphasis	mobility

1 Stand tall with your feet apart, knees soft. Reach up from the top of your head to the ceiling to check that your back is correctly aligned. Keeping your right arm by your side, pressed lightly against the leg, breathe in and lift your left arm in front of you and slightly to the side.

2 Keeping the ribcage still, start to draw a circle with the arm as you breathe out. If the ribcage moves, you are swinging too far—move the arm farther away from the body to the side and draw a smaller circle. Imagine that you are drawing on the wall to the side of you with your fingertips.

3 Complete the circle, trying at all times to keep a slow, consistent speed. Imagine a wheel turning, with continuous motion and no sudden jolts. When you have completed 10 circles on one arm, change arms and repeat.

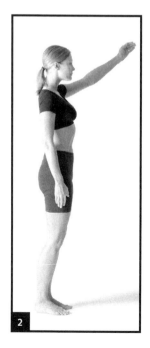

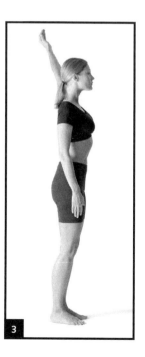

double-arm circles

reps	10 times
visual cue	arm hoops
emphasis	mobility

1 Stand tall with your feet apart, knees soft. Start with your arms slightly in front of you. Keep your abs pulled in and check that your back is in alignment.

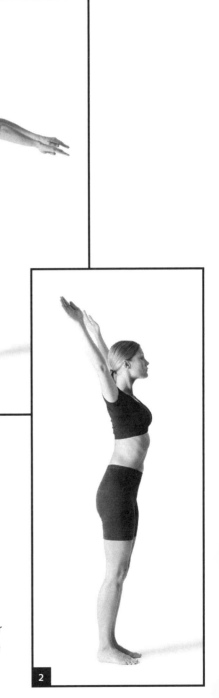

1

2

2 Breathe out slowly and circle both arms back. Try to keep your hands together as you reach to the ceiling. Make sure that your back does not arch by keeping your abs pulled in as tightly as possible. Keep the speed of your movement constant and try to increase the size of the circle. When you reach 10, repeat in the opposite direction.

toy soldier

reps	10 times
visual cue	air paddle
emphasis	mobility

1 Stand tall with your feet apart and knees soft. Breathe in. Reach your left arm to the ceiling and your right arm to the ground.

2 Breath out as you bring the lifted arm forward and down, swapping to lift the lower arm up to the ceiling. Keep your torso still and stretch the top of your head to the ceiling. Keep the speed slow and the action smooth. Repeat 10 times.

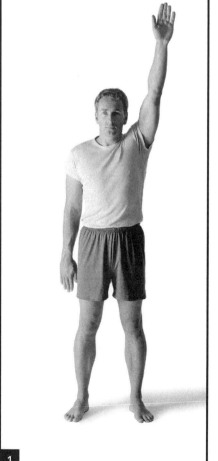

1

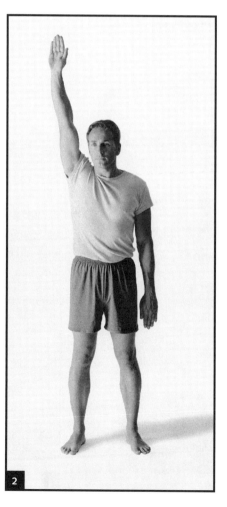

2

WORKOUT

foot stretch

It's best if you do this move with your shoes and socks off.

■ CAUTION

Make sure that the surface you are leaning against is strong.

reps	5–10 breaths each side
visual cue	pushing a car
emphasis	shin stretch

1 Stand facing close to a wall. Bend your left knee and step back with the right foot. Tuck the right toes under as you breathe out, then press into the wall lightly and bend the right knee a little farther. Push down on the top of the foot to stretch this area. After 5 to 10 breaths, switch legs.

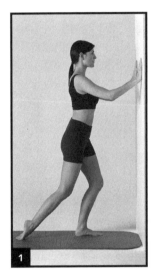

58

WORKOUT

runner stretch

To increase the stretch, move the front leg a little farther forward, then lean farther into the movement.

■ CAUTION

Practice this move in front of a mirror to ensure that the knee and foot stay in line. If your weight pushes forward over the front knee, this can cause discomfort in the knee joint.

reps	5–10 breaths each side
visual cue	straddling
emphasis	stretch

1 From a kneeling position, lunge forward with your left leg until your knee and foot are in line—you should feel the stretch in the inner thigh of your right leg. If you don't feel it, slide the left leg farther back until you do. Place your hands on either side of the left foot with the left toes pointing forward.

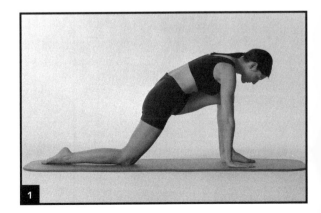

runner stretch

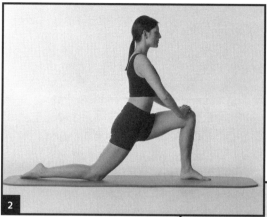

2 As you breathe out, lengthen the upper body so that you lengthen the spine into a neutral position. Place the hands on the left leg, just above the knee joint.

3 In order to advance the stretch, float the right knee off the floor on your next outbreath and place your hands next to your left foot to stabilize you. Check that the front knee and ankle are in line.

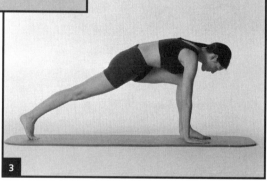

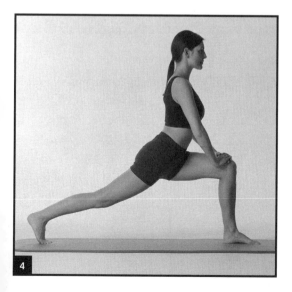

4 On your next outbreath, lengthen the upper body so that you extend the spine into a tall, neutral position, and place the hands on the front leg, just above the knee joint. Hold the stretch for 15–30 seconds; try to increase this time as you become familiar with the movement. Switch legs and repeat.

hamstring stretch with dynaband

You can use a towel if you don't have a dynaband.

▮ CAUTION

Don't lock the knees and don't force the stretch.

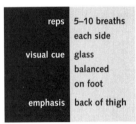

reps	5–10 breaths each side
visual cue	glass balanced on foot
emphasis	back of thigh

WORKOUT

1 Lie on your back, knees bent and feet flat. Bring your left foot up toward you and wrap the dynaband under it. Take a firm hold of the band with both hands, and as you breathe out, lengthen your left leg toward the ceiling. Keeping your leg straight and your elbows tucked in, pull gently on the band to draw your leg closer to your chest. Concentrate on maintaining a neutral spine as you do this.

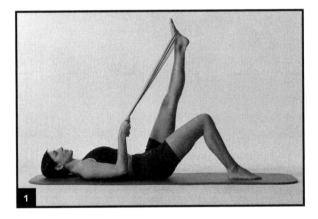

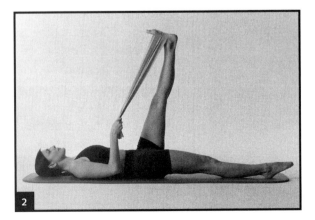

2 To challenge yourself further, as you breathe out lengthen your right leg along the floor, flexing your foot. Again, concentrate on maintaining a neutral spine.

quad stretch

**Pull the leg gently back—
don't force the knee.**

█ CAUTION

*If you feel any pain in your
knee, stop at once.*

reps	5–10 breaths each side
visual cue	hopscotch
emphasis	front of thigh

1 Lie in a line on your side, maintaining a neutral spine.

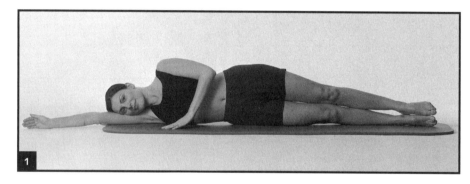

WORKOUT

2 Reach out with your left hand to take hold of your left foot, keeping your hips and knees stacked on top of each other. Gently push your foot into your hand. Add a little resistance to this move by using your hand to draw your foot closer to your butt. You should feel the stretch in the front of your thigh as you do this.

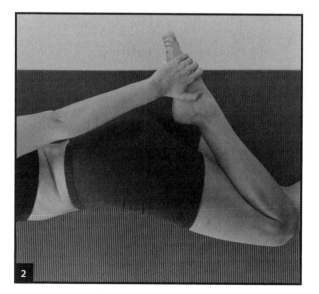

seated spine stretch

Think of the movement as a single, long, slow sequence. Be careful not to strain your back, and try to keep all your joints in neutral alignment.

reps	5–10 times each side
visual cue	leaning over ball
emphasis	mobility

WORKOUT

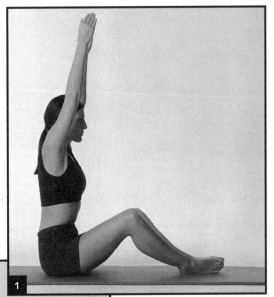

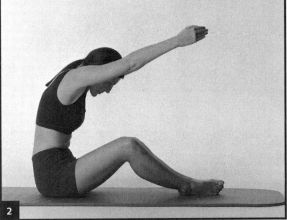

1 Sit tall in a neutral position with your feet hip-width apart and your knees relaxed. Raise your arms so that they are pointing straight above your head. Breathe in. As you breathe out, draw in the lower abdominals toward the spine.

2 Slowly bend forward, rolling the spine down as you do so. Lead with your head, let the chin drop to the chest, then allow the shoulders to roll over and the weight of the arms to carry you down as far as possible without losing control. Relax and gently bend the knees as you curl down to the floor. Pay attention to your hips; if you feel that they are pushing out behind you, bend your knees more, and don't go as low. You should feel as if you are folding into yourself.

chest stretch with ball

If you don't have a ball, you can use a chair instead.

█ CAUTION

Don't lock your elbows— keep them soft. Never force a stretch.

reps	5–10 breaths
visual cue	bowing on knees
emphasis	stretch

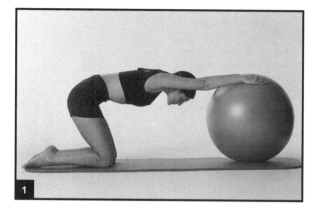

1

1 Kneel in front of the ball. Place your hands onto the ball, shoulder-width apart. Try not to have the ball too far away, otherwise it will feel unstable. As you breathe out, keep your hands on the ball, and sit your butt back toward your heels. Your butt doesn't need to touch your heels—just sit back far enough to feel a stretch through your chest muscles.

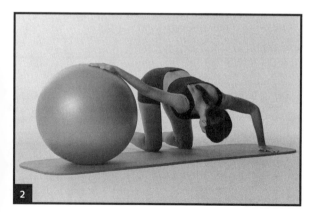

2

2 To stretch the upper part of your chest, kneel alongside the ball. Take your left hand out slightly wider than your shoulder, and put the right hand onto the ball. Breathing out, gently drop the right shoulder toward the floor. As you do this, try not to rotate from the hips, just the right shoulder.

hip rolls

The movement should be continuous, but pause briefly in the center before rotating in the opposite direction. Allow the rate of your breathing to control the speed of the movement.

reps	5–10 times each side
visual cue	child rolling
emphasis	strength and mobility

1 Begin by lying on your back with your knees bent, your feet flat, and your arms open in a crucifix position. Draw your shoulders back and down, and rotate your head to the left, in a position where there is no tension in the neck. Keep your legs bent and your knees together as you breathe out, and slowly allow the knees to roll to the right side. You don't have to touch the floor with your knees, but rather rotate to a position where the knees can stay together and where there is no tension or pinching in the lower spine. As you breathe in, bring the head and legs back to the center position. On the next outbreath, rotate the head and legs in the opposite direction.

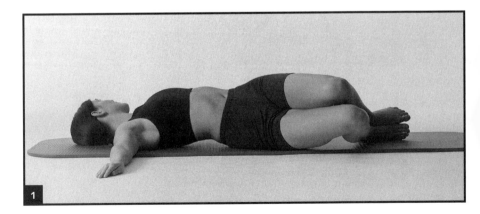

1

hip rolls

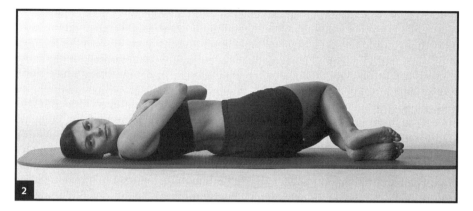

2 This variation is the same as stage 1, but with both arms crossing the chest so that the hands are touching opposite shoulders. Maintain this position as you rotate your legs and head in opposite directions.

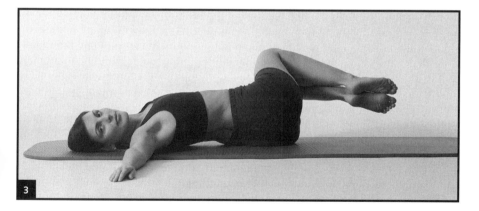

3 Once you have mastered the first two positions, try this more challenging version. Lift your feet off the floor, keeping the feet and knees together, and rotate your legs to one side as you turn your head to the other.

the saw

This movement works on the mobility and stretch of your upper back.

! CAUTION

Do not force the stretch. Take it to the point of tension and relax to allow the final push. Do not struggle to complete the move. If touching your toes proves difficult, build up to it slowly.

reps	10 times
visual cue	plane propellor
emphasis	mobility

1 Sit with your legs hip-width apart and your feet flexed. Lift your arms on either side of you. They should not be open too wide, just enough so that you can see them as you look forward. Lift your head up as though you are in a movie theater and trying to see over someone tall.

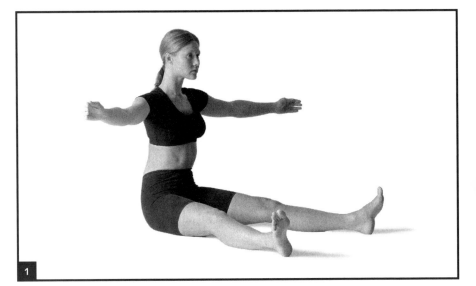

1

the saw

2 Breathe out and turn your body to the left side. Keep your arms in line with your shoulders as you turn. Do not let them cross the body. Turn equally to the back and side, keeping your hips facing firmly to the front.

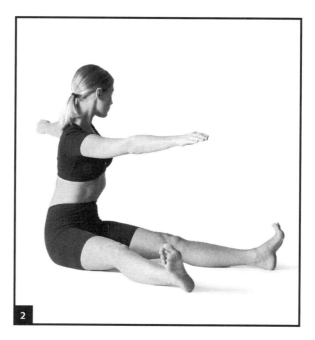

2

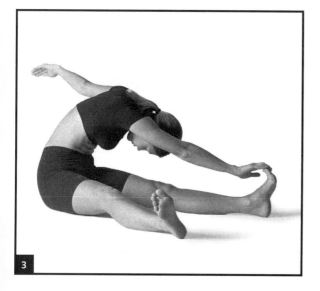

3

3 Continue to breathe out as you stretch your right hand to your left foot to the point of tension. Imagine you have a large beach ball over your knee and that you are stretching over it. Keep your head down as you stretch. Breathe in as you come back to the center and repeat in the opposite direction on the other side.

strength & stretching

These exercises are at the core of the Pilates technique. Each balances stretching with strengthening; many offer an "as you get stronger" variation. It's fine to challenge yourself but don't exceed your comfortable range of movement.

the hundred

As you move your legs, brace your center to keep firm support. Keep both hips level as you lift your leg.

❚ CAUTION

Remain focused on keeping your body in the neutral position. Check that the size of the arch in your lower back has not increased or decreased as you lift and lower your leg.

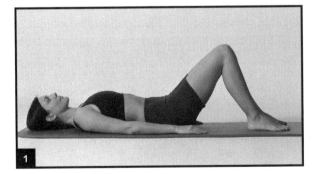

reps	10 times each side
visual cue	steep slope
emphasis	abdominal strength

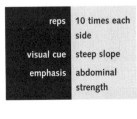

1 Lie on your back with your knees bent and your feet flat on the floor, comfortably close to your butt. Find the neutral position and, with your arms by your side, draw the shoulders back and down. Imagine that there is an orange between your chin and chest, and try to lengthen through the back of the neck.

the hundred

2 As you breathe out, lift the left leg to form a right angle, checking that the knee comes directly above the hip and that the foot is in line with the knee. Hold this position for five breaths, keeping your hips braced. On the fifth outbreath, lower the leg to the start position. On the next outbreath, lift the other leg and repeat the movement.

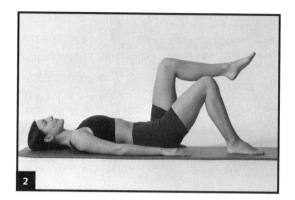

as you get stronger

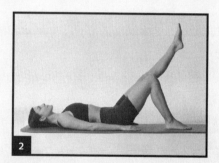

2 To challenge yourself further, lift your leg off the floor while at the same time lengthening it. Because the weight of the leg has been increased, you will need to focus on maintaining your neutral position. If you lose the position, lower the level.

3 Once you master the above level, try the hundred with both legs lifted. Lift one leg as in stage 2 above, and imprint your lower spine into the mat. Lift the second leg, and allow the spine to return to neutral. Hold for five breaths, focusing on not letting the ab muscles dome or the lower spine come out of neutral. On the last breath, lower one leg at a time, and return to the starting position.

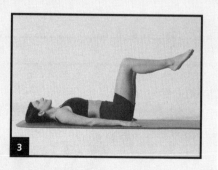

swimming

Imagine you have a piece of paper passing under your abs. Try not to touch it with your stomach. Find how high you can move without letting your abs touch the mat.

▌CAUTION

Keep elbows soft. There should be no pressure in the lower back. Do not hunch the shoulders.

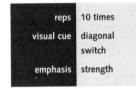

reps	10 times
visual cue	diagonal switch
emphasis	strength

1 Lying face down, stretch the top of your head forward and slide your shoulders down your back. Stretch your legs behind you, keeping them hip-width apart, and contract your abs to lift your navel off the floor. This is the position you must try to maintain throughout the movement. Isolate the upper body by keeping both legs down. Breathe out as you lift your head and right arm up and away from the floor. Breathe in as you lower your arm and then change to the left. Your goal is to keep your navel off the mat.

2 Isolate the lower body by putting your head on your arms in front of you. Slide your shoulders down your back. Breathe out as you lift the right leg away from you. Tighten the stomach and lift off the floor. Lower the right leg and change to the left.

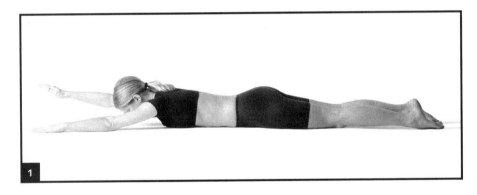

1

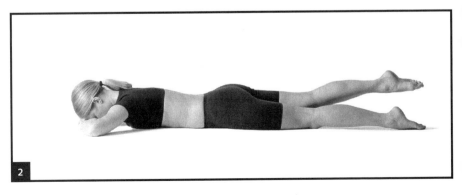

2

as you get stronger

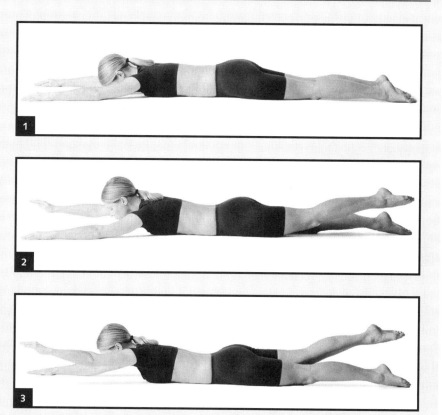

1 Lying face down, stretch the top of your head forward and slide your shoulders down your back. Stretch your legs behind you, keeping them hip-width apart, and contract your abs to lift your navel off the floor.

2 Breathe out as you lift your left leg and right arm up and away from you. Lift your limbs as high as you can without touching the mat with your navel. Feel your muscles lengthening along the floor before you lift. Do not struggle to lift too high because the lengthening is more important.

3 Breathing in, lower the limbs to change to the other side. Your little finger and little toe should be on the same diagonal line in space. Keep the movement slow and controlled. The speed of the movement should stay the same on both the lifting and the lowering of your limbs.

push-up

Focus on this as a long, continuous single movement.

❗ CAUTION

Soften or bend the knees if necessary: if your hamstrings or lower spine are tight, soften these areas more before you start.

reps	5–10 times
visual cue	snail on wall
emphasis	strength

1 Stand tall in the neutral position with feet hip-width apart and shoulders drawn back and down. Imagine your eyes are looking over the horizon, and take a breath in to prepare for the movement.

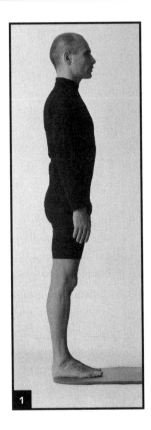

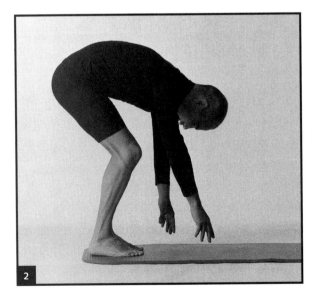

2 As you breathe out, begin to roll your head and spine downward, starting from the neck. Imagine each vertebra is in a chain that is moving link by link. Allow the weight of your arms to carry you forward.

push-up

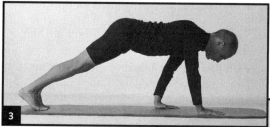

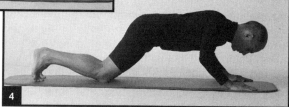

3 As you reach toward the floor, breathe in and bend your knees to enable your hands to touch the floor. As you breathe out, walk your hands along the floor until they are directly below the shoulders with your back level; keep your butt in line with your shoulders.

4 Slowly lower your knees onto the mat without causing any impact to your knee joints. Now walk your hands forward two paces. Realign the shoulders over the hands to create a slope from the hips to the knees. Keep this alignment as you do the push-up. Work back slowly through the positions until you come back to the standing position.

as you get stronger

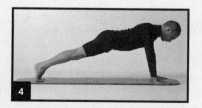

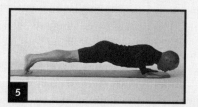

4 Follow stages 1 to 3. Your hands should be directly under the shoulders, your shoulders drawn back and down away from the ears, your neck relaxed, and your eyes looking toward the floor.

5 Keeping the neutral alignment, breathe in and lower your body. Draw the shoulders back and down, trying to keep the back in neutral and your butt in line with your shoulders. Go as low as you can without losing the correct body alignment. Work back slowly through the positions until you are back to standing.

rolling back

Be patient and gentle with your spine until you feel that rolling becomes natural and you can return to the seated position with ease.

reps	10 times
visual cue	hedgehog
emphasis	mobility

1 Sitting tall, lift from your center, imagining a taut string connecting the crown of your head to the ceiling. Bend your legs and place your feet together, flat on the floor. Use your hands as supports with palms down, close behind you. Pull in your stomach muscles

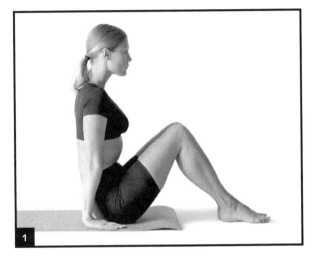

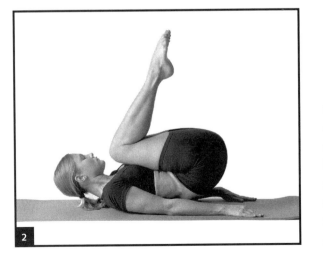

2 Breathe in as you tilt your pelvis and gently roll back. Use your arms to support your weight as much as needed while, on the out-breath, you roll up again. Be sure to keep your abs contracted.

as you get stronger

1 Place your hands on your shins and pull in your stomach muscles.

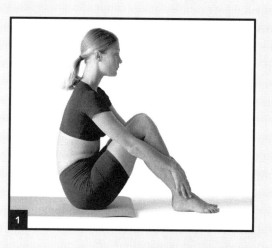

2 Taking a slow breath in, curl your pelvis and start the roll, with your chin near your chest and spine curled.

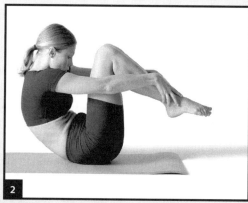

3 Gently roll back only as far as your shoulders. As you roll back up, with abs still contracted, begin to breathe out slowly. Complete the breath as you return to the seated position and lengthen your spine to the ceiling. Aim to make the roll as smooth as possible.

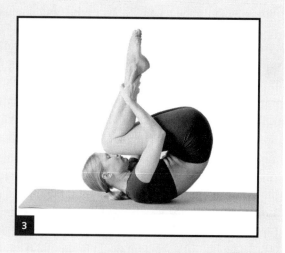

roll-up

Imagine that your spine is a chain or a system of links: each area of the spine should work independently as you work through the movement to create a smooth, chain-like movement.

█ CAUTION

Keep your feet on the floor, and avoid spurts of speed as you roll up: the move should be smooth and continuous.

reps	5–10 times
visual cue	the morning sun rising
emphasis	abdominal strength

1 Lie on your back with your legs straight and your arms stretched over your head. Draw your shoulder blades back and down.

2 As you breathe out, begin to peel your head and shoulders off the floor, and slowly lift your arms toward the ceiling as you come up.

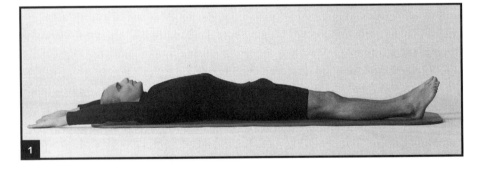

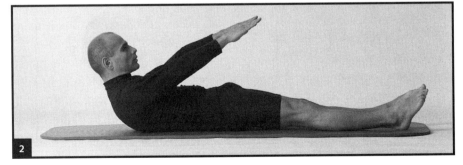

roll-up

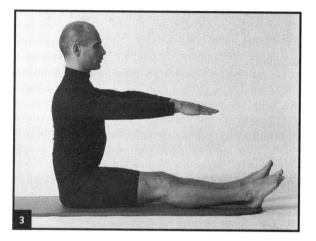

3 Continue to roll forward slowly, peeling your spine off the floor vertebra by vertebra. Roll through the pelvis until you reach a sitting position.

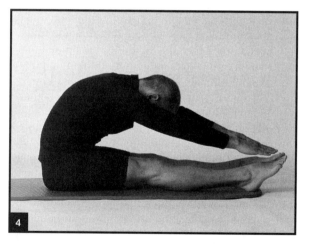

4 Breathe in as you lengthen out over your legs, stretching your arms toward your toes as far as you feel comfortable. As you breathe out, reverse the move and slowly lower your body back onto the mat: begin by rolling through the pelvis, then roll down vertebra by vertebra.

swan dive

As you breathe in, lower your body back down to the floor. Allow the speed of your breath to control the speed of the movement, which should be continuous.

reps	5–10 times
visual cue	lying on thin ice
emphasis	spine mobility

1 Lie on your front and open your arms out on the floor, aligning your elbows with your shoulders. Make half a rectangle shape with your arms and draw your shoulders back and down. Keep your eyes looking down and your neck in line with your spine. Breathe in to prepare, and as you breathe out, float your chest away from the floor. The move should be small, so try not to focus on lifting the whole chest. Your elbows and hands should stay in contact with the floor: use them to push gently into the floor as you lift, but focus on lifting with the muscles in your back rather than those in your arms.

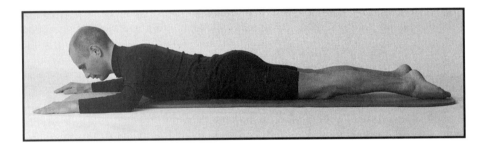

modification with ball

Kneel in front of a large ball, and curve your body over it. Place your hands behind your head with your elbows out wide and create a "tabletop" with your back and neck, not letting your head drop over the ball. As you breathe out, lengthen and lift your chest away from the ball, not allowing the ball to move underneath you. Remember that the movement should be small and controlled.

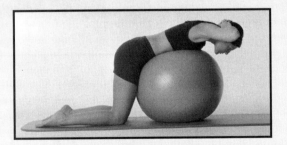

as you get stronger

Try to relax your glute muscles (butt). If you clench them, they will help to stabilize you as you lift. The focus should come from your abdominals and back instead.

1 Starting from the lying position, place your arms by your sides with the palms touching your sides. Draw your shoulder blades back and down.

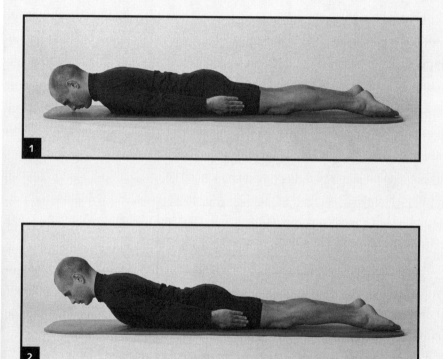

2 Breathing out slowly, float your chest away from the floor. As you breathe in, lower it again. Lift with the muscles of the back in the thoracic area. As you lift, lengthen the muscles in the lower part of the spine. If the muscles in the lower back are tightening or pinching, then relax down and rest, or return to the variation using your arms (see page 74).

hip circles

Aim to keep the spine in neutral while doing this movement. Also try to keep the distance equal between the knees and chest as you rotate from side to side. The movement should be smooth and continuous.

reps	5–10 times each side
visual cue	wheel
emphasis	strength

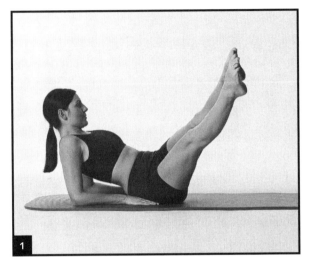

1 Rest on your elbows, lifting your chest to the ceiling, and try to maintain a neutral spine. Bend your knees as you breathe in, and breathe out as you lengthen your legs.

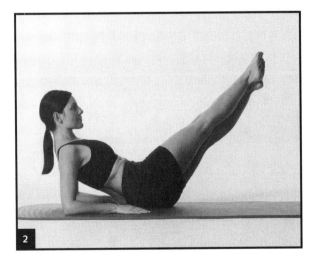

2 Swing your legs around to the left side, holding your position at the top of the movement. Repeat to the right side.

WORKOUT

as you get stronger

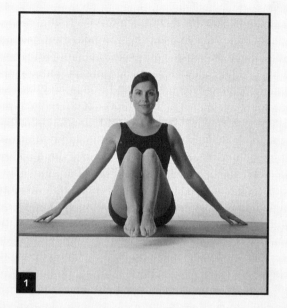

1 Sit tall in a balanced position with your feet comfortably close to your butt. Your hands should be out to the sides in a balancing position, and your feet and hands should only lightly touch the floor.

2 As you breathe out, lift your legs straight up in front of you, then swing your hips to the right; as you breathe in, swing back to the center. On the next outbreath, swing to the left, and continue from side to side.

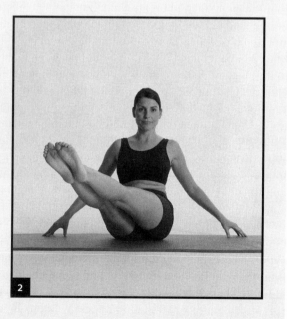

one-leg circles

The main movement is the circling of the knee, but try also to focus on the top of the thigh circling within the hip joint as if it were drawing a smooth circle inside the joint. Don't let the weight of the leg drop heavily into the hip joint, and try to keep the hips level and in the neutral position.

reps	5–10 circles each way, each side
visual cue	clock
emphasis	mobility

1 Lie on your back, with knees bent and feet flat on the floor comfortably close to your butt. Find neutral, and with your arms by your side, draw the shoulders back and down. Imagine an orange between your chin and chest, and lengthen through the back of the neck.

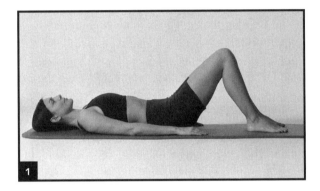

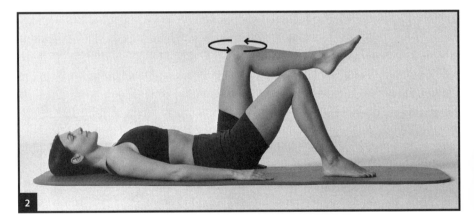

2 As you breathe out, lift the left leg to form a right angle: the knee should be directly above the hip and the foot should be in line with the knee. Keeping the left knee bent, draw a small circle on the ceiling with the knee, ensuring that it remains directly above the hips. As the knee comes in toward the center of the body, breathe in; as the knee travels away from the body, breathe out. Perform five circles in each direction, trying to increase the size of the circle slightly with each motion. Once you have drawn five circles in each direction, breathe out and slowly lower the leg to the starting position. Repeat with the other leg.

WORKOUT

as you get stronger

This advanced movement opens up the hip joint, increasing mobility.

▌ CAUTION

If your hips move, you are taking the rotation too wide. You may find that each side has a different range of mobility. Limit your movement to the range allowed by the least flexible hip and keep the leg motion smooth. This will eventually restore balance to both hips.

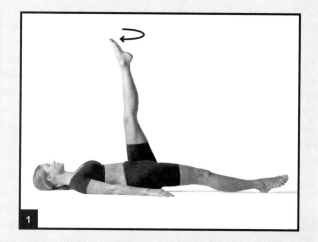

1 Lie relaxed and flat on the mat with your arms at your sides and palms down. Pull in your abs. Pointing your toes, stretch the left leg to the ceiling as far as possible without straining. Maintain a neutral spine (page 37). Rotate the left leg clockwise, using the hip joint as the center of the clock face. Breathe in from 12 to 6 o'clock and breathe out from 6 to 12 o'clock.

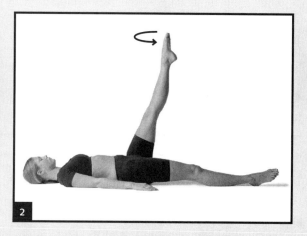

2 Repeat counterclockwise, breathing in from 6 to 12 o'clock and breathing out from 12 to 6 o'clock. Switch to your right leg and repeat.

side lifts

Progress through these moves over a period of sessions. Doing them all in one session will exhaust the areas of your body being worked.

▮ CAUTION

Allow your body to lift itself to a position where it is challenged, but is not straining.

reps	5–10 times each side
visual cue	rocking
emphasis	leg and butt strength

1 Lying on your right side, lengthen your legs, keeping your heels in line with your hips (if your feet are behind your hipline, you may feel lower back discomfort). Stack your shoulders, hips, knees, and feet on top of each other. Relax your head onto your lengthened right arm, and draw your right waistline away from the floor. Place your left hand on the floor just in front of you, and draw your shoulders back and down. As you breathe out, lift the top leg. Then, as you breathe in, lower the leg within an inch of the bottom leg, before raising it again on the next outbreath. To advance these moves, try to lift both legs on the outbreath and lower them on the inbreath. Keep the legs a few inches off the floor until you have completed the sequence. Then lower the legs to the floor.

2 As a further challenge, take the front hand off the floor and stretch your arm along your side.

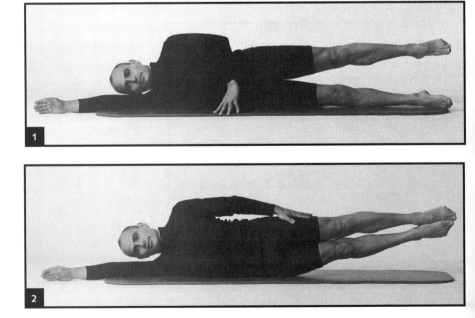

as you get stronger

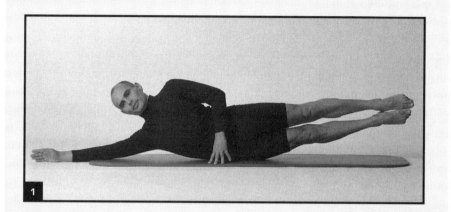

1 Once you have mastered the basic moves, try lifting the upper body on the outbreath at the same time as lifting the lower body. For extra stability, place the top hand in front of you.

WORKOUT

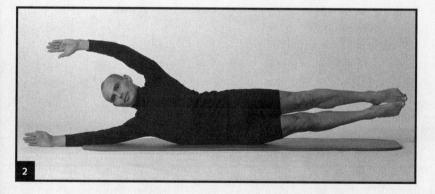

2 Now try to lift your upper body and lower body, lengthening the top arm over your head on the outbreath. As you breathe in, lower the head back to the bottom arm, the top arm back to your side, and the legs about an inch off the floor.

shoulder bridge

This movement is for opening and mobilizing the whole spine.

❗ CAUTION

Do not force this movement. Be very gentle with your spine. If you know you have tightness in a certain area, then slow down as you pass through it. Concentrate on gently coaxing your muscles into becoming flexible.

WORKOUT

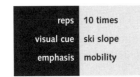

reps	10 times
visual cue	ski slope
emphasis	mobility

1 Lie on your back with your arms by your side. Keep your arms beside you on the floor throughout this exercise. You may use them to help you stabilize, but avoid gripping the surface of the floor with them. Think of the top of your head pulling you to one end of the room and your tailbone stretching to the other. Breathe in to prepare, keeping your center strong.

2 Breathe out and start rolling up toward the ceiling, leading with your tailbone, letting your vertebrae lift one by one from the mat. Lift your hips up, taking them to the height where your body forms a slope, no higher.

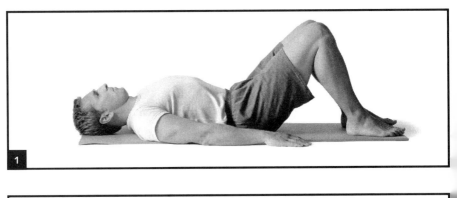

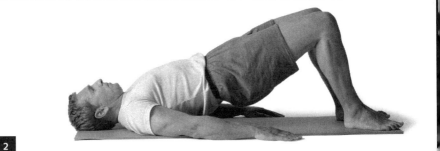

shoulder bridge

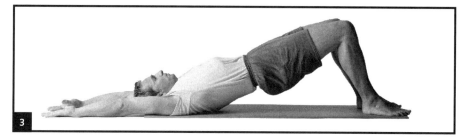

3 At the top of the movement stretch your arms behind you and breathe in. As you breathe out start rolling down back to the mat as if laying a string of pearls on a piece of velvet. Visualize each vertebra as it touches the mat.

as you get stronger

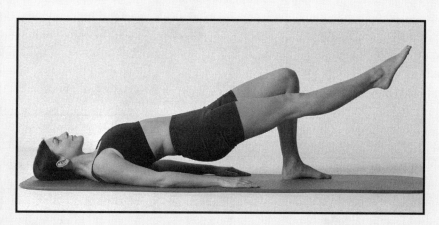

3 An advanced option is to add the leg and balance movement. Keeping your arms by your sides, slowly peel the spine up to the shoulder bridge position. Brace your hips, and on your next outbreath, unfold your right leg and lengthen it to the ceiling. Breathe in as you lower the leg to restabilize and breathe out to lower the spine back down to the floor. Repeat with the left leg.

the seal

This rolling exercise is more advanced than the rolling back movement (page 74) but also creates mobility and flexibility in the spine.

❚ CAUTION

If you find this movement too difficult, return to the basic rolling back exercise in which you may use your arms to support yourself.

WORKOUT

reps	10 times
visual cue	rolling ball
emphasis	mobility

1 Take a balanced position holding your legs lightly. Lift the top of your head to the ceiling and contract your abs.

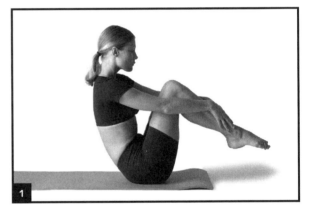

2 Breathe in as you roll back onto your shoulders. Stay in a tight ball. As you roll, imagine that you are imprinting your spine into the mat.

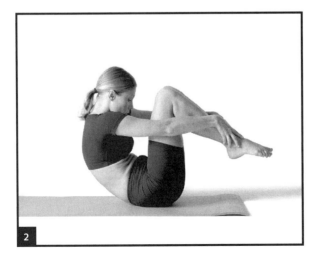

the seal

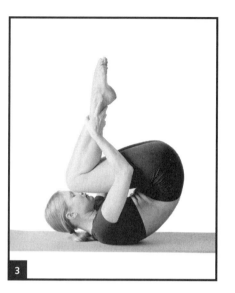

3

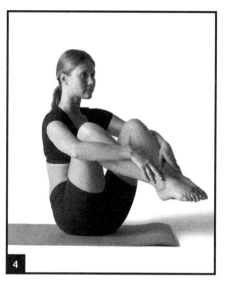

4

3 Breathe out as you come back up and return the roll to the seated position. Use the muscles at your center to power yourself back into the balanced position.

4 At the balanced position, lift the top of your head to the ceiling and gently pull your legs apart then push them back together in three beats. Check that your spine is as straight as possible.

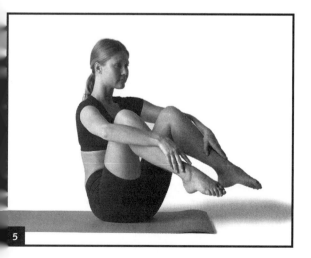

5

5 This beating of the feet adds to the balance period and also increases the strengthening element of the movement. Focus on your center and imagine it is initiating the pull. The strength for the balance position should also come from your center.

glossary

Abdominal muscles (abs): the muscles layered across the midriff that lie across each other at various angles. There are four types: the rectus abdominals, internal obliques, external obliques, and transversus abdominals.

Aerobic exercise: any sustained activity that works the heart and lungs, increasing the amount of oxygen in the blood.

Alignment: arrangement in a straight line.

Cardiovascular: relating to the heart or the blood vessels.

Centering movements: the Pilates exercises that work the center of the body, abdominals, and back.

Core exercises: the Pilates movements that concentrate on strengthening the abdominal and back muscles.

Crunching: sit-ups where the abdominals are not engaged so much as squeezed together, shortening the space between the hips and ribcage.

C-shape: the shape of the spine when the body is slumped over and bent due to bad posture.

Elongation: lengthening of the muscle. Leaner muscles develop from stretching the muscle rather than bulking it up.

Hidden stress: when muscle groups compensate for an injury or difficulty by using larger muscles to protect weaker ones.

Hyperextension: extending further than 180 degrees. Hyperextension occurs when the muscles tense up and the elbows or knees lock, resulting in a reverse bending.

Imprinting: gently pushing each vertebra into the mat, as though it were leaving an indentation.

Lumbar curve: the bend of the spine at the small of the back.

Neutral spine: the spine in its most natural position, which might not necessarily feel comfortable or "normal."

Overloading: point where the effort required by a muscle to withstand an applied weight is too great. The tissue may tear or rupture as a result.

Powerhouse: the name that Joseph Pilates gave to the abdominal area, found between our ribcage and hips.

Pilates exercises work this area in order to create a stronger, more balanced lower back.

Prone: lying facedown.

Resistance: an opposing force that pulls in the direction opposite to the one created by your muscle.

Rolling: exercises where the spine rolls over the mat, one vertebra at a time.

Soft knees: holding the knees relaxed and slightly bent, rather than locked.

Supine: lying down on the back.

Tendon: elastic linking tissue that connects bone to muscle.

Tripod position: where the feet support the body weight by distributing it evenly over three points: the ball of the foot, the middle of the heel, and the outside edge of the foot, near the little toe.

Vertebra: one of the bony segments that make up the spinal column.

Visualization: use of mental imagery to aid the accomplishment of physical tasks—an important element of the Pilates technique that helps the mind more effectively control the body.

GLOSSARY

index

Names of individual movements are indicated in **bold** type

A

abdominal breathing, 24
abdominal muscles
  balance 1 52
  balance 2 53
  breathing 24
  centering 26–29
  hip circles 80–81
  hundred, the 68–69
  one-leg circles 82–83
  roll-up 76–77
  seal, the 88–89
  shoulder bridge 86–87
  side lifts 84–85
  swan dive 78–79
  swimming 70–71
arms
  chest stretch 54
  double-arm circles 56
  one-arm circles 55
  push-up 72–73
  swimming 70–71
  toy soldier 57

B

back
  hip rolls 64–65
  muscles 24
  neutral spine 28, 37–39

pain 17
roll-up 76–77
rolling back 74–75
round back (the cat) 48
saw, the 66–67
seal, the 88–89
seated spine stretch 62
shoulder bridge 86–87
spine swing 51
standing spine twist 50
swan dive 78–79
swinging 49
balance 1 52
balance 2 53
balancing the body 7, 9, 16, 42–43
breathing 10, 23–24
butt
  shoulder bridge 86–87
  side lifts 84–85
  swimming 70–71

C

the cat (round back) 48
centering 26–29
chest stretch 54
chest stretch with ball 63
clock technique 39
concentration, development of 10, 20–21

control 31
core, the 24, 26
cross-training 12

D

double-arm circles 56

E

equipment 10

F

foot stretch 58

G

goals, setting 14–15

H

hamstring stretch with dynaband 60
health, impact on 7, 12
hip circles 80–81
hip rolls 64–65
history of Pilates 9
hundred, the 68–69

I

injuries, preventing 16
isolation of muscles 42–43

K

kyphosis posture 35

L

lateral breathing 23–24

legs
  hamstring stretch
    with dynaband
    60
  hip circles 80–81
  one-leg circles
    82–83
  quad stretch 61
  runner stretch
    58–59
  shoulder bridge
    86–87
  side lifts 84–85
  swimming 70–71
lordotic posture 35

M
muscles 16, 24
music 20–21

N
neutral spine 28, 37–39

O
one-arm circles 55
one-leg circles 82–83

P
pain, preventing 16
pelvic floor 24
  activating 28–29
Pilates, Joseph 6, 7, 9,
  14–15, 26
plumbline test 35
posture 6–7, 12,
  34–35
  adverse symptoms
    of poor posture
    34–35

unbalancing
  muscles 16
powerhouse, the 26, 32
precision 40
push-up 72–73

Q
quad stretch 61

R
roll-up 76–77
rolling back 74–75
round back (the cat)
  48
runner stretch 58–59

S
saw, the 66–67
seal, the 88–89
seated spine stretch
  62
shoulder bridge
  86–87
side lifts 84–85
spine see back
spine swing 51
**standing chest
  stretch** 47
standing spine twist
  50
stress, reducing 21
stretching
  chest stretch 54
  chest stretch with
    ball 63
  foot stretch 58
  hamstring stretch
    with dynaband
    60

quad stretch 61
round back (the cat)
  48
runner stretch
  58–59
seated spine stretch
  62
spine swing 51
standing chest
  stretch 47
standing spine twist
  50
swinging 49
wall stretch 46
swan dive 78–79
sway-back posture
  35
swimming 70–71
swinging 49

T
tai chi 32
thoracic breathing
  23–24
toy soldier 57

V
Valsalvic method
  breathing 24
visualization 31–32

W
wall stretch 46
warm-up exercises
  46–53

Y
yoga 10

other Ulysses books

ASHTANGA YOGA FOR WOMEN:
INVIGORATING MIND, BODY, AND SPIRIT WITH POWER YOGA
Sally Griffyn and Michaela Clarke, $17.95
Presents the empowering practice of power yoga in a balanced fashion that addresses the specific needs of women.

HOW TO MEDITATE: AN ILLUSTRATED GUIDE
TO CALMING THE MIND AND RELAXING THE BODY
Paul Roland, $16.95
Offers a friendly approach to calming the mind and raising consciousness through various techniques, including meditation, visualization, body scanning for tension, and mantras.

THE JOSEPH H. PILATES METHOD AT HOME:
A BALANCE, SHAPE, STRENGTH & FITNESS PROGRAM
Eleanor McKenzie, $16.95
This handbook describes and details Pilates, a mental and physical program that combines elements of yoga and classical dance.

PILATES PERSONAL TRAINER BACK STRENGTHENING WORKOUT:
ILLUSTRATED STEP-BY-STEP MATWORK ROUTINE
Michael King and Yolande Green, $9.95
The easy starter program in this workbook teaches Pilates exercises that are appropriate for strengthening the back in a safe and healthy manner.

PILATES PERSONAL TRAINER POWERHOUSE ABS WORKOUT:
ILLUSTRATED STEP-BY-STEP MATWORK ROUTINE
Michael King and Yolande Green, $9.95
Designed for those who want to flatten and shape their abs, this book explains each Pilates exercise in an easy-to-follow manner. The key element is the series of two-page, step-by-step photo sequences that illustrate and demonstrate each exercise.

PILATES PERSONAL TRAINER THIGHS & BUTT WORKOUT:
ILLUSTRATED STEP-BY-STEP MATWORK ROUTINE
Michael King and Yolande Green, $9.95
Instead of paying $100-plus per hour for private Pilates sessions, those looking to get the same kind of targeted workout to shape and slim their thighs and buttocks can find it in this book.

PILATES WORKBOOK:
ILLUSTRATED STEP-BY-STEP GUIDE TO MATWORK TECHNIQUES
Michael King, $12.95
Illustrates the core matwork movements exactly as Joseph Pilates intended them to be performed; readers learn each movement by following the photographic sequences and explanatory captions.

PILATES WORKBOOK FOR PREGNANCY:
ILLUSTRATED STEP-BY-STEP MATWORK TECHNIQUES
Michael King and Yolande Green, $12.95
Presented in an easy-to-use style with step-by-step photo sequences of Pilates matwork techniques—adapted here for pregnancy and post-pregnancy.

SENSES WIDE OPEN: THE ART & PRACTICE OF LIVING IN YOUR BODY
Johanna Putnoi, $14.95
Through simple, accessible exercises, this book shows how to be at ease with yourself and experience genuine pleasure in your physical connection to others and the world.

YOGA IN FOCUS: POSTURES, SEQUENCES, AND MEDITATIONS
Jessie Chapman   photographs by Dhyan, $14.95
A beautiful celebration of yoga that's both useful for learning the techniques and inspiring in its artistic approach to presenting the body in yoga positions.

YOGA FOR PARTNERS: OVER 75 POSTURES TO DO TOGETHER
Jessie Chapman   photographs by Dhyan, $14.95
An excellent tool for learning two-person yoga, *Yoga for Partners* features inspiring photos of the paired asanas. It teaches each partner how to synchronize their movements and breathing, bringing new lightness and enjoyment to any yoga practice.

OTHER ULYSSES BOOKS

To order these books call 800-377-2542 or 510-601-8301, fax 510-601-8307, e-mail ulysses@ulyssespress.com, or write to Ulysses Press, P.O. Box 3440, Berkeley, CA 94703. All retail orders are shipped free of charge. California residents must include sales tax. Allow two to three weeks for delivery.

about the authors

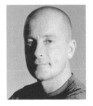

With more than two decades of experience in Pilates, **Michael King** first started working with the Pilates technique while he was a dancer at the London School of Contemporary Dance. He trained with Alan Herdman, the first teacher to bring Pilates to the United Kingdom from the United States. In 1982, he opened his own studio in London. Two years later, Michael moved to Texas, running a studio for the Houston Ballet Company while training in the new Fonda-established aerobics. Michael is the company director of the Pilates Institute, the United Kingdom's leading Pilates training company.

Yolande Green has been an instructor in the fitness industry for more than a decade, teaching aerobics, step, spinning, body conditioning, and Pilates. She is currently studying for an M.Sc. in health and fitness. Yolande is the company director of the Schools' Fitness Advisory Service, a training company for exercise teachers in secondary schools, and also serves as a presenter and tutor for the Pilates Institute. She has run many successful exercise and education groups, and has given presentations at fitness conventions and workshops around the world.

acknowledgments

Many thanks to all the instructors and staff at the Pilates Institute, not only in London but also in the many other countries that continue to promote the work of Joseph Pilates through our name. This book is dedicated to our great friend and colleague Sarah Irwin, who continues to be a great inspiration to many Pilates Instructors both here in the U.K. and in the U.S. where she lives.

—Michael King

I hope that this book enables people to learn and utilize the Pilates technique in the same way that I have. I would like to thank Michael for his time and mentoring and to acknowledge the support received from my Mum and Dad and my boyfriend Pete.

—Yolande Green